ALSO BY JAMES COOK

Memory Songs

IN
HER
ROOM

IN
HER
ROOM

HOW MUSIC HELPED
ME CONNECT WITH MY
AUTISTIC DAUGHTER

JAMES COOK

Published by Lagom
An imprint of Bonnier Books UK
Wimpole Street
London
W1G 9RE

www.bonnierbooks.co.uk

Hardback 9781788701860
eBook 9781788701877

A CIP catalogue of this book is available from the British Library.

Designed by Envy Design Ltd
Printed and bound in Great Britain by Clays Ltd, Elcograf S.p.A.

1 3 5 7 9 10 8 6 4 2

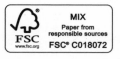

Every reasonable effort has been made to trace copyright holders of material
reproduced in this book, but if any have been inadvertently overlooked the
publishers would be glad to hear from them.

Lagom is an imprint of Bonnier Books UK
www.bonnierbooks.co.uk

Some names, identifying details and locations have been changed.

For Emily

Contents

PART II:

Age 22 months to two-and-a-half years

PART III:

Age two-and-a-half to three

'One of the last great realisations is that life will not be what you dreamed.'

James Salter – *Light Years*

PROLOGUE

Walking On Sunshine

Sardinia, July 2011

I'M SITTING IN the passenger seat of a hired Toyota Yaris. Outside the windows, scorched wheat fields, motionless olive groves; sparse, low buildings flash past. The motorway is deserted, and through the open sunroof I can see the noonday sky, a deep unblemished blue. In the driver's seat is my girlfriend of ten months, Anita. Whenever I think of her – us – I feel a surge of intense happiness. We are in the first flush, the first glorious phase.

I open a heavy bottle of mineral water and offer her a sip. She takes one tanned hand off the wheel and tips it to her lips. Then, with a smile, gives it back.

'Thank you,' she says, the trace of a German accent, her wide grey eyes on the ribbon of tarmac ahead.

'Shall we stop at this beach? Costa Rei.' I ask, squinting at the well-worn map on my knees.

'Yeah, why not.'

We take the next slip road.

It is the end of our first holiday together. Three hours earlier, we packed our tent, parasol, defective Primus stove and suitcases into the boot of the Yaris, and prepared to leave the tree-shaded campsite. After checking that no rubbish had been left, Anita headed off to the modest *supermercato* that we'd come to know well during our short stay. I waited by the car, sunlight slanting through fragrant pines; and from somewhere, scents of eucalyptus and rosemary, too. The air was cool, but another day of blazing heat was ahead. Moments from the past week returned: meals and beaches, road trips and conversations. Our in-jokes and catchphrases, well honed now. We seemed to thrive on humour. We'd never had an argument, which was a good sign, surely. The first holiday was meant to be a test, an audition for future compatibility. We'd shared a tent, so ... perhaps we could share a house some day? A life?

And then I spied her, smiling, walking that singular, sashaying walk of hers, with a surprise in her hands: two takeaway coffees. She thought of everything.

Sardinia had been my idea. An obsessive James Bond fan as a boy, I knew *The Spy Who Loved Me* had been filmed here in 1976. Driving along the coastal roads, every terrifying hairpin (with rugged mountains on one side and the glittering ocean on the other) was *that* car chase, the one with the white Lotus Esprit. But we were not, alas, in a white Lotus Esprit. In fact, the modest vehicle from Holiday Autos and the flights had been an enormous financial stretch for me, an ex-indie band songwriter in my early forties, who still earned a precarious living as a musician in London. But I wanted to make a gesture. Show her I was serious.

We'd met when I was at work. I carried a mental snapshot of her at this moment – small, ash-blonde, captivating smile. She was over a decade younger than me, and came from a small town near Frankfurt. When I asked what she did, she said she was planning on becoming a primary school teacher in the UK, but at the moment was a teaching assistant, looking after a challenging autistic boy who bit and scratched. I recall admiring the calm way she talked about it; how it bespoke reserves of grit, yet revealed a sensitivity, too.

And then we lost touch. Many months later, a text out of nowhere, a series of dates, and now I'm in a car on a sunlit Mediterranean island with her, in love.

The radio is tuned to an Italian pop station. 'Walking On Sunshine' by Katrina and the Waves comes on. The eager drum tattoo; the triumphant, leaping brass; the ardent, breathless vocal that contains a perceptible note of victory – *I've found the one* – mirror my own feelings. We haven't talked about it yet, but I've been wondering what we'd be like as a married couple (that's if she was crazy enough to say yes).

We enter a big, empty car park bordered by dense woodland. When we come to a halt, I unclip the seat belt and open my door. The sudden siege of heat is tempered by a robust breeze, and I can hear a tremendous noise of wind and waves from just behind the trees. The air has that fresh marine smell – salt and the iodine tang of seaweed, triggering a rush of excitement remembered from boyhood holidays. I go to the rear of the car and open the boot, search around for different shorts, more-suitable footwear. When I close the door, I see that Anita is waiting, ready with beach bag over her shoulder, the parasol under her arm, and a stylish, colourful seventies headscarf over her hair.

'Come on!' she says. '*Milk Sticks.*' Her endearing name for my white, un-tanned English legs. That smile, mischievous now.

We make our way through dunes and scrubland, finally reaching a dilapidated wooden path partially submerged by drifts of white sand. The wind buffets my ears, a huge assault, like the roar of a jet plane. We must be very near the ocean. Then, rounding a bend, we are met with an astonishing sight. Costa Rei, extravagantly wide and empty, sweeping for bright kilometres in both directions. The sea, far-off, is greenish blue, in constant wild motion: breakers exploding on the shoreline, and further out, new waves building. Above the horizon, the sky fades up from a pale duck-egg blue to a deep, rich navy. The only structure, about a hundred metres away to our right, is a wooden hut on stilts. A red flag – *Danger, No Swimming* – flaps madly above it. I imagine I can make out the slumped, sleeping figure of the coastguard.

We both start laughing. This is unbelievable. The whole beach to ourselves! I start to film the scene on my phone. Anita races to the shoreline, shrinking to a toy-like figure; throws her hands above her head, then runs back, girlishly sticking out her tongue to the camera. A strand of blonde hair has broken loose, fluttering in the wind. We walk on until we find a sheltered spot in the dunes, where we plant the parasol, lay out our towels and sit staring at the distant ocean as it roils and rages. The light. The sand – deep and warm and fine in texture. The invigorating air … What a find, this beach, I think to myself, on our last day; a moment of pure grace to mark the end of what has been the best holiday of my life.

I notice Anita is rubbing the toes of her left foot, pulling and massaging the skin. An injury from earlier in the week.

'Here, let me kiss it better,' I say, leaning over, momentarily aware of the infantilising nature of the phrase, and hoping I haven't said the wrong thing.

'You'd make a good dad,' says Anita.

I freeze.

Would I? No one has ever said that before. The question of parenthood has been much on my mind recently, for there is something else we haven't talked about yet. Something which began as a vague notion, a wish, that has now become a deep aspiration. A crazy dream. Perhaps, one day, we'll have a child.

Part I

Age 11 to 21 months

1

In My Room

Surbiton, September 2015

FOUR YEARS LATER, and the dream has come true. Anita and I are married, with an 11-month-old daughter, Emily.

We live in a Victorian conversion, a building that is something of a rarity on our street. Apart from a similar house next door, the road consists of a variety of 1930s bungalows, Art Deco residential courts, and the 1960s blocks typical of Surbiton. We are on the top floor, the servants' quarters (aptly enough, for parents of a young child). At some stage in the flat's life, an architect removed the low ceilings and transformed every room into a set from a James Bond film. This, of course, was the reason I wanted the place so badly, when we viewed it over a year before. A mezzanine has been installed. There are gantries and a steel ladder. High, sliding doors, all in white. A large aquarium-style fish tank set into a cambered wall, where one would expect to find the severed hand of an unfaithful assistant, or some Siamese fighting fish at the very least. In the main bedroom are fitted wardrobes that cover an entire wall, mirrored with Ken

Adam-style roundels, not un-like 007's fridge in *Goldfinger*. A pad, basically. Not a child-friendly home. Tiny fingers could become caught, or worse, in those heavy doors. Indeed, after a while, a Heath Robinson aspect to some of the alterations becomes apparent. The doors don't work smoothly, constantly overlapping or getting stuck. The bathroom, almost entirely made of wood, is slowly rotting away, and spares no longer exist for the fittings after the local firm that manufactured them closed down.

The flat has the least cost-efficient energy profile it's possible to have. Heat escapes merrily through the old, ill-fitting sash windows (something the architect didn't change), a fact that concerns me about Emily's room, which is boxy, lined with bookshelves, and dominated by a large IKEA cot. Worse, the old wooden floors disclose lethally sharp nails during warm weather. And the treacherous, rusting fire escape that leads to the garden is a Health and Safety inspector's dream. So perhaps it wasn't an architect who converted the place after all, but merely a Bond fan who had a go. Whatever the story, it is definitely not somewhere to raise a child. But then we didn't know we were going to have a child when we moved in. Three days after we did, to our surprise and delight, Anita's pregnancy test showed positive.

It helps to know that the landlords are a couple with a young family. They lived in the flat safely for ten years, but apparently became bored with the place. Now we are the unremunerated custodians of their ever-inflating asset. They won't even meet us – all dealings with them are conducted through the letting agent.

Despite this, I love the flat. It is easily the best place I have lived in London (and we are still in London – Surbiton hasn't been part of Surrey since 1965), a city I've been renting in for close on 30 years.

On Tuesdays and Wednesdays, I take Emily to a nearby nursery, 8:00am to 1:00pm. Anita has gone back to teach part-time at a primary school, leaving me in charge of our daughter on Mondays. This split arrangement suits me fine – I still work as a poorly paid musician in the evenings, playing guitar and singing in a chain of jazz and blues clubs, while finishing my first book, a memoir about nineties music, in the days when Anita is at home.

The lounge window is where Emily and I conduct our Monday vigils, her warm weight curled against my shoulder. I point out the birds that perch in a tall copper beech tree: feral parakeets, an extraordinarily vivid lime green in colour. Or single magpies, which we must salute. (The maintenance of this particular superstition is backbreaking: we can see up to 20 a day.) Beyond the tree is the gentle elevation of Church Hill Road, pleasingly foreshortened like a television cricket pitch, which leads the eye to the spire of St Mark's.

When we tire of the lounge, we move to the main bedroom window. Here, the view plunges down to well-maintained back gardens, all except one – with unruly grass and a dilapidated shed that is slowly being engulfed by ivy – which is ours. On the better-kept lawns, blackbirds peck at fallen crab apples. More magpies hop and flap (*One for sorrow, two for joy, three for a girl, four for a boy*). And above, a line of tall plane trees with overlapping crowns that seem to form a single canopy, where acrobatic squirrels leap from bough to bough. Beyond this, the wide channel of Claremont Road. I count red buses for Emily, flashing by between houses: a swift block of colour, then the empty street again. And in the distance, to the west, the un-prepossessing spire of St Andrew's church, and the pale lights of Heathrow. To the east, looking towards Richmond, a strange flat-topped cedar with a crown like a crooked pointing finger. I tell Emily that a giant walking from Richmond became tired and he sat down on the tree. Now it's a sign that shows us the way to Kingston upon Thames. How I look forward to inventing stories for her, when she's older.

When we tire of the bedroom we move back to the lounge. Sometimes I play Beatles or Pink Floyd songs for her on guitar, which she seems to like. Or we watch cyclists zip by in hi-vis gear; the postman with his scarlet trolley; the pensioner in the block of flats across the road, sitting in her lounge all day watching television, her perm as white as a cauliflower in the gloom. Peace. Quiet. Ennui. Despite the Bond-ian nature of the flat's design, it's hardly exciting, our sleepy Surbiton life.

Emily – an October baby, a Libran – is rapidly approaching her first birthday. Already, her character is emerging: happy, sweet and affectionate, yet spirited and vivacious, too. And what's more, she's beautiful. Heart-stoppingly beautiful. A pinched, button nose, startlingly clear blue eyes, sandy hair that bears hazel highlights in the sunshine; flawless skin. A Renaissance cherub. I know all parents think this about their children, even the ones that resemble hammerhead sharks, but she really is an exceptionally good-looking child. I lose count of the people –

other parents, strangers in the street – who say, 'Gosh, she's a pretty one!' or, 'So photogenic!' or, 'What a bonny lass!' I'm used to these remarks now, as we parade down Claremont Road, Emily strapped in the buggy. Street cleaners, schoolgirls, office workers, pensioners – all of them are drawn to her, compelled to look down and return her striking, spontaneous smile. It's practically a public service we're offering. I realise I'm showing her off – *look at what my genes have produced.*

But Emily's beauty carries worry, too. Madeleine McCann-esque abduction scenarios assail me. (This is actually whom she resembles most: Madeleine, the poor stolen child with the perfect blonde hair; the big, trusting, other-worldly eyes.) Once, back in the summer, in a Rye pub, an ageing all-day drinker passed us on his way to the door. Staring at Emily – who was smiling up at him from her pram – he cackled: 'It's all right, darlin', I just want to nick you.' I still shudder at the memory.

Yet, despite these fears, we're enjoying being Emily's parents; feel blessed to have her in our lives.

One of these anxieties is that Emily seems to cry much more than other children her age. Since her birth – a fraught, 33-hour labour followed by a forceps delivery – she's suffered from colic reflux, a chronic digestive complaint that causes severe abdominal pain. She screamed almost constantly at first – a six-month Extreme Noise Terror gig – the memory of it an exhausted, grey blur. The colic improved over time, but a seemingly causeless tendency towards crying remained. Emily is a paradox among her NCT group peers: the baby that smiles the most, and the baby that cries the most.

On nursery mornings, I leave the house with the buggy at 7:30am, the September air brisk, planes on the Heathrow flight path crossing the cobalt blue sky. Office guys with rucksacks and well-groomed women making their way to the imposing Art Deco train station. And me in my new-dad uniform of porridge-stained fleece and trainers; Emily in her cream coat with the heart-shaped buttons, her red felt hat fastened under her chin.

As we walk, she tips her head back, looks up, and I study her eyes as she absorbs the fast-moving stream of images passing by. Sometimes I imagine I glimpse fugitive reflections in them: the spears of railings, blackbirds in flight; tree branches, the tips of their leaves just turning yellow. Or a jet plane making its way overhead, leaving chalky traces on the blue. She's taking in the world. I wonder what she is thinking. She doesn't have any words yet, and the rest of her development is slightly behind her contemporaries. At 11 months, she isn't crawling, and we've told the nursery that she has balance issues: she can sit up, but will keel over eventually. They need to be vigilant.

Yet we're not too worried about any of this. Emily is just a late bloomer, that's all. Her engaging, adorable nature overrides these shortcomings. She's alert, quick to laugh; delighted to be alive. Staring down at her, I wonder if she will always be as sweet and charming as she is now. She doesn't seem to have any of the child's natural meanness in her. That is all to come, perhaps – after the age of two, 'the drop' as *Peter Pan* author J.M. Barrie called it. He claimed that this marked the end of innocence.

*

One afternoon, sitting in the high-windowed living room with Emily, I'm struck by how fascinated she is by the circular mirror on the pea-spattered playmat. Everything is new to her, especially her own reflection. *Hello, you*, I imagine her thinking. *I find you oddly pleasing, strangely compelling.* I make a mental note to keep a diary of all her milestones and discoveries over the coming year. Like most parents, I don't want to miss anything. I want to be there for Emily's first attempts to crawl, her first steps, her first word.

A record is playing on the turntable, the Beach Boys' 'In My Room'. We nearly always have music on, or I will play those Beatles' and Pink Floyd songs for her on the guitar, during our days together. It feels good to have an excuse to sing and play outside of work, and it seems to calm Emily when she's upset.

As the Wilson brothers' numinous Californian voices fill the lounge, I begin doing something I often do idly on hearing a favourite tune: try to calculate how many times I must have listened to it. And how many times there will be left. I'm 46 … Then, suddenly, I realise an uncomfortable truth. Nothing is new for me anymore. I've come to the end of music.

The only artists I listen to – if I listen to anything at all – are the old faithfuls, the trusty stand-bys. The canon. *BeatlesBeachBoysMarvinJoniBowieZep*. OK, satisfaction is guaranteed, but isn't it a bit, well … predictable? Much like always choosing the same dish in a restaurant. A commonplace middle-aged ossification – something I always said would never happen to *me* – has set in. I'm pushing 50. Emily is about to turn one. If everything is new for her, why can't it be for me, too?

It was a gradual leave-taking, a decade or so of falling musical testosterone levels. If I'm honest, pop just doesn't affect me like it used to. It feels like it has all been done before, and far better, decades previously. I've stopped buying albums by new artists. The only CD purchased in the last year has been Led Zeppelin's re-mastered *Physical Graffiti*. I don't even buy *Mojo* magazine anymore.

Like Emily, I decide it's time to face the future fearlessly. I resolve there and then to download Spotify. Investigate those up-to-the-minute bands with implausible names, obscure song titles, pretentious lyrics. *Beards*. Even some of the old artists I've tried over the years, but never managed to fully embrace. The Neu!s and the Beefhearts and the Steely Dans. Give them a proper listen at last.

And then a whole plan comes to me. For a year – from Emily's first birthday to her second – I will consume only new music, while keeping a record of her development. I won't be allowed to listen to anything that is already in my collection: all that stuff will be banned, perhaps even physically locked away. It seems like the perfect solution, the cure for a slightly clichéd early mid-life malaise. True, much of the new music might be like drinking cod liver oil, but I will feel virtuous, and perhaps even shake off the soul's sleep. And the marvellous thing is I will have an accomplice, someone to help keep my spirits up during the dark days when I just want to listen to the Beach Boys. I glance at Emily. She is right there in front of me, gazing out of the window, after losing interest in her own smiling reflection. She will be on a voyage of discovery, too.

We can even sit and play the latest sounds together, this jaded ever-hopeful listener, and the insatiably curious one-year-old. By the end of the year, will I have regained my passion for pop? Consume rock again with renewed intensity? Or will I conclude that I was right all along, that everything has already been done?

And one last thing: I set myself another task. I want to learn a different language, German, over the coming year (we're raising Emily to be bilingual). It will be necessary, and a useful exercise, too, attempting to master new skills at the same time as my daughter. I want to know what that is like at such an advanced age. I also want to know what they are saying about me, behind my back.

So I raise a toast to my record collection, and to Emily: here's to a year of new discoveries, just the two of us together.

2

Running Up
That Hill

IN THE WEEKS before Emily's first birthday, I binge on Kate Bush records, immersing myself in the work of one last canonical artist before I start to look for all the new stuff. The album I play the most is Kate's masterpiece, *Hounds of Love*, released 30 years ago this month. How many records issued today will still be listened to 30 years hence? I wonder. The LP is frontloaded with the hits, and what strange hits – commercial melodies that are not trying to be commercial. Music that just *is*; music that has to come out.

More than any other artist I can think of, Kate Bush's oeuvre embodies the mysterious realm of childhood. Not just the early Eden of innocence (captured on 'In Search Of Peter Pan' from her second record, *Lionheart*), but the next stage: the conflicted emotions and fear of puberty that surface at around the age of ten, explored on *The Kick Inside* and *Hounds of Love*. On the latter album, Kate sings in character as a little girl, frightened of the dark; traumatised by finding a wounded fox in the countryside, after which she runs away, leaving it to die ... A childhood spent on the edgelands, where town meets country. This was my childhood, too; one spent running through the fields and woods that bordered Hitchin, the quiet Hertfordshire market town where I grew up.

Hounds sets me off on a mental expedition, back to the past. I find the videos for the hits on YouTube. In the comments thread below 'Running Up That Hill' someone has written: 'This is my eighties childhood. This is looking at my mum and dad from my car seat.' Likewise – except, for me, Kate Bush inhabits the seventies. I try to remember when I first became aware of her: 1978 most probably; 'Wuthering Heights', the startling debut on *Top of the Pops*. I would have been nine, my parents recently separated. I recall the teachers chatting about her performance at school the next day; first break, instant coffee on their breaths. Mine was a fairly laid-back, progressive primary, and this sort of gossip wasn't unusual to overhear from the bearded fellows and cheesecloth dress-wearing women who taught us. They seemed as mildly shocked as I was. Who was this strange singer with the intense, imploring stare, waving her arms above her head like a dervish? She looked tiny in the video – it was hard to tell as she was alone, there was no way to gauge scale – but this only added to her kinetic power. It was this image that lingered the following morning, but also the name 'Cathy'. We had a family friend called Kathy, and it seemed oddly right that she should be in the song (intriguingly, she also appeared in Simon and Garfunkel's 'America'). Even better, 'Wuthering Heights' mentioned the moors – I spent parts of my childhood in Yorkshire, visiting my stepfather's mining town, so the song seemed to have been written specially with me in mind.

One of the teachers compared Bush to the eccentric new wave singer Lene Lovich, citing her high-pitched voice. I knew this was wrong – Kate was far classier. Yet despite the hippy-ish dress she wore in the video there *was* something punk-like, rebellious, about Bush. Blondie's 'Denis' was in the chart at the same time, and in my mind I filed Kate Bush alongside Debbie Harry. Both women projected a similar vitality, a fearlessness.

A few years passed, and Kate Bush seemed to fade from view. Her videos seldom appeared on *Top of the Pops*. Then, suddenly, in 1985, she was back. Several lifetimes seemed to have elapsed since Kate last appeared on television, but here she was again, with a smash-hit album of childhood-tinged songs about discovering wounded animals, burying yo-yos in the garden, the wonder of big skies and cloudbursts. My favourite track on *Hounds of Love* was 'Cloudbusting', the video for which always seemed to be on *The Tube*. Apparently, the song was *un hommage* to *A Book of Dreams*, a memoir by Peter Reich, written for his father, Wilhelm Reich, a doctor and Freudian psychoanalyst. Reich Snr had designed a 'cloudbuster', a steampunk contraption that caused rain when pointed at the sky. In the video, Bush, playing the young Reich, and Donald Sutherland, acting the role of the dad, haul the machine up a hill on a gauzy summer's day. The hill always put me in mind of Hitchin's Windmill Hill, a place where my twin brother and I used to fly kites. Behind this, the tune's rising, hopeful string part, repeated endlessly over a military drum tattoo lends the scene a hypnotic quality. Yet it is the lyric that ensured the song became my favourite from the album. Kate insists, over and over again, that something good is just about to happen …

Many years – and many London lifetimes – later, it is the 'Cloudbusting' video I play the most on my YouTube excursions into Kate Bush nostalgia, long after Emily has gone to sleep. The song has a different, deeper meaning, now that I'm a father. *It's you and me, daddy*, sings Kate, at one point. It sets in motion a train of thought about the parent-child relationship. What does it mean to be a father? What do I want for my daughter? What will she make of me? In the video, the boy believes his dad can perform miracles, draw rain from the heavens. My ego is flattered by the idea, but I think I'd settle for just being a good teacher. I'd like to show Emily all the beauty and magic in the world – not in a naff, man-splaining way, I hope – but in the same spirit you might excitedly present a friend with a book or an album. That's my naïve aspiration, anyway.

So what *do* I want for my daughter? What are my hopes for her? These are selfish questions (What do *I* want), but every parent has them. I want her to have an archetypal happy childhood, each year looking forward to Christmas in a warm, cosy book-lined house with an advent calendar; eating chocolate from the tree, and sniffing the pine needles. (A scenario that Kate Bush captures perfectly in 'December Will Be Magic Again'. Not the song itself – a slightly directionless piano ballad – but the *title*.) I want her to ride a bike and build a snowman. I want her to have a brother or sister. I want her to love music, and maybe learn to play an instrument one day. I want her to practise ballet, play football, ride a horse, enjoy judo or gymnastics. I want her to go shopping for clothes and make-up with friends; go camping or travelling with them, experience freedom. (But not too much freedom …) I want her to have a career that she loves. I want her to marry: a man or a woman, I don't care which. I just want her to be happy.

Out in Surbiton with Emily one crisp, late-September morning, a young woman passes us. Blonde, small, no more than 20; stylish black pea coat, brown autumn boots; chin up, walking with purpose somewhere. All the freshness of youth in her face. Her whole life ahead of her. In moments like these, I always wonder if this will be my daughter some day. What job will she be doing? Will she be a doctor? (The passer-by looks like our GP, Dr Daly.) I try to picture Emily as a young woman, happy, ready to take on the world.

Who will she be?

*

The lounge. A Monday. Emily is sitting quietly on her playmat, staring up at the shimmering crown of the copper beech tree outside the window, communing with it. I'm watching her, marvelling at the astonishing perfection of her face, when she notices me, and we both start laughing. She smiles at me in real recognition, I think, for the first time, and a bright flame of tenderness for her suddenly blazes in my heart. Nobody tells you it's possible to feel this much love. Well, they do, all the time, but nobody can tell you what the experience actually feels like.

Later, Anita and I decorate Emily's room with giant, colourful wildlife stickers. I put up a giraffe first, which doubles as a height-measuring device. Soon there are trees and clouds, monkeys and vines. An entire jungle. Finally, I hang a print illustration of a lion from a children's book, in tribute to Kate Bush: *Emily the Lionheart*.

This is the room in which I will read her bedtime stories. I can't wait until she's old enough to become lost in the same fabulous tales that I had read to me by my father as a boy: *Charlie and the Chocolate Factory*, *Alice's Adventures in Wonderland*, *A Bear Called Paddington*. (Before she was born, I bought her a hefty *Roald Dahl Treasury*. Each time I passed a charity shop I plundered it for books: *The Gruffalo*, *The Moomins and the Great Flood*, old Ladybirds.) So far, I've tried reading her the Mr. Men and Little Miss series, with varying degrees of success. She won't sit still, or swipes the book away, and rarely looks at the pictures. When she does listen, I try to imagine what she's thinking: *Come on, roll your sleeves up, put some elbow grease into it. I want voices, actions, ad-libs, but not too many, stay faithful to the text …*

I can't wait until she can speak.

A friend – a father of two – said to me: 'It gets so much better when they start talking; they become "people". You get something back.' When I told him that Emily hadn't spoken any words yet, he said, 'Oh, she will. It's all about to get really interesting.'

*

One Sunday towards the end of September, Anita and I walk by the river to Kingston with Emily in the pram. Our daughter leans forward, eager to see the geese on the towpath; fascinated by the ever-changing patterns of the water. It's mild, and sunshine dazzles us. A strong, almost maritime breeze blows.

On the sparkling Thames, small boats with blue sails work in formation. When we've seen enough, we head back to Surbiton, and Long Ditton recreation ground, an unremarkable playing field on the border with Seething Wells. At the far end, the elevated railway line runs: trains with their red, yellow and blue SWT insignia surge past every few minutes, a torrent of sound containing odd ghost notes.

The rec incorporates the most popular kids' play area in town, and is usually overcrowded on Sundays, but despite this we queue patiently for the swings. When at last it's our turn, we hoist Emily up into the little caged seat. It's the first time she's been on a swing. I'm suddenly moved by her enjoyment. She loves the motion, the reckless feeling of freedom. Her tiny, smiling face zooms in; we push her away, then back she comes. 'We'll go on the slide next!' I say. 'Then we can try the roundabout!' Her life is just beginning, I think to myself, a sea of possibilities lie ahead. An odd phrase formulates in my mind: *You can have a bit of everything, my darling. Think of life as a feast – you can have a bit of everything.*

When we return to the flat, I cook an actual feast – chicken and roast potatoes with thyme, rosemary and lemon; red and green peppers, leeks, onion gravy – and afterwards, with the plates still un-cleared, I sing 'Row Your Boat' for Emily while bobbing her on my knee.

Row, row, row your boat,
Gently down the stream,
Merrily, merrily, merrily, merrily,
Life is but a dream.

I feel a vast contentment, a deep, profound happiness. We are a family, a trinity, a completion. A three-piece. It was always my favourite band line-up; the intuitive closeness, everyone on their parts. Once, when I was 40, single and childless, living in another part of Surbiton, I recall looking down from my flat window to the courtyard below and seeing a young couple play with their little daughter. They were spinning her around and around for no other reason than it made her happy, and it made them happy, too. As I watched, and listened to their laughter ring around the open space, I felt a sharp stab of envy, and of grief, almost – *I'll never have this.* And yet here I am – here *we* are – in the house where Emily, in her cramped room with its jungle stickers and lion print, will dream her first dreams. I'm a family man. And tomorrow, we will spin Emily around and around, and laugh and laugh.

September becomes October. The season is turning, slyly, to autumn. I give the tangled lawn its last mow before winter. On cold nursery mornings, I change and dress Emily in the orange-curtained half-darkness of her room – she still can't sit up for long, so removing her pyjamas and putting on new clothes has to be done with her perched on the edge of the waist-high changing mat, steadied by my free hand. By now, she helps find the ends of sleeves by raising her arms. I sing the Beatles' 'I Wanna Hold Your Hand' when I see the tips of her delicate fingers emerge. I'm careful not to snag one. (A lesson I have learned, dressing or carrying a small child: never rush.) To pull her trousers up, I must stand her on her feet. She leans her head on my shoulder, like a drunk taking a leak in an alley.

Eventually, she's dressed: olive-green dungarees and a bright red top. All buttons, no poppers: the sure giveaway sign that the clothes, due to financial necessity, are hand-me-downs. But, like her mother, she looks fabulous in anything.

Steam issues from boiler flues as I barrel down Church Passage, the wide cut beside the house, Emily strapped in the buggy. My thumbs freeze on the handles. Breath *shrrs* out in front of me. Just the thinnest patina of frost visible on car rear windows. When we arrive at the nursery, Emily's tiny nose is as red as her top. I wipe two green candles of snot from above her lip, and fireman's lift her to the door. We always seem to be the last ones. Her playmates, sitting around the low breakfast table, meet my eyes with their customary neutral expressions, their level evaluating stares. I've always found the nerveless scrutiny of toddlers discomfiting … But as I hand my child over to the key worker's welcoming arms, Emily's cry of joy reassures me that everything will be all right.

I take the river road back. The sun is low and rising behind the workmen's cottages. A cloudless sky. Tiny comets – vapour trails – climb. My heart is beating fast; I have an obscure feeling of imminent Good News, as if some wonderful gift is waiting for me just around the corner. 'Cloudbusting' is in my head – something good is about to happen. I make my way up Westfield Road, directly into the sun, past the terraced houses, past a neglected canary-yellow Lotus Eclat that's always been parked there, and walk with purpose along St James's Road. Then out on to Claremont. The scene looks like something the Canadian Tourist Board might have cooked up: hectic reds, glowing golds, ochres, taupes. The chestnut trees are exploding into their autumn finery. Conkers, shiny as coins, fall heavily onto the roofs of parked cars. Winter will soon be here. Christmas. December will be magic again! I realise I can't remember a time when I've been more excited about the future – everything seems charged with meaning.

It's all about to get really interesting.

3

The Rainbow

FOR EMILY'S BIRTHDAY, we spend a week in Gran Canaria. The last days of October. It's not a holiday from hell exactly, but neither is it an experience I'd like to repeat in a hurry. We are with some new friends of ours: another couple, Andrew and Carrie, and their irrepressible 16-month-old son, Billy. They are not the problem – more sanguine, convivial travelling companions I could not imagine. No, the problem is Emily. She hates the holiday, absolutely *hates* it. I'd say at a conservative estimate, the ratio between her crying and not crying is 80:20. Sometimes more. Is it the heat? The change of surroundings? The fact that she is recovering from a cold? The view from the bedroom window not good enough? I'll never know: she can't tell me. It's deeply upsetting, and I try everything possible to ease her distress.

When the crying becomes really dreadful (and I lose count of aborted trips to restaurants and beaches), I walk her around on my shoulder, singing to her. It's the only activity that brings calm. I do this most evenings, lingering at the back of the villa, where there is a sort of garden, and the temperatures are lower. 'Row Your Boat', 'Ticket To Ride', 'Across The Universe', 'Old MacDonald', 'The Wheels On The Bus', 'Blackbird', 'Yellow Submarine', the Peppa Pig theme (*Duh, duh, duh, duh – duh, duh, duh, duh, duh, duh*), anything to stop the noise. She stares up into the blue night, reaches out towards trails of scarlet and purple bougainvillea, touches the cool Canarish slate of the wall, and there is peace. But I know the racket will begin again, the moment we step back indoors.

So I do what any Englishman abroad does, whether facing adversities or not: drink. Not on my own, of course. I have help – from Andrew, principally. By the end of the week, the pile of bottles waiting to be collected by the recycling van is shamefully large. We're almost certainly in line for some sort of award from the Gran Canaria local council.

A few days in, we decide to visit the mountainous region in the centre of the island. It will be cooler there, and perhaps more pleasant for Emily. We rent a dodgy-looking Dacia, with a single rusting windscreen wiper, and a leaking air-conditioning unit. At least that's what the fellow at the car hire place says it is. Hopefully it isn't brake fluid …

The weather is warm and dry when we set out – the four of us, plus babies – cramped into the tiny seats, driving slowly up winding roads, Andrew manfully at the wheel. I sit in the front with him. We pass huge cacti with bulbous orange flowers, and, in the distance, on the craggy rock face, we spot tiny cave mouths, and miniature waterfalls. Palm trees appear in the lush valleys. There's excitement at all this, but I'm not having a good time. I've forgotten that I'm not great on snaking mountain roads, with plunging, heart-in-the-mouth sheer drops of many thousands of feet to certain death on either side. My knuckles whiten on every bend. To make matters worse, Emily howls in the back, while Anita, suffering from car sickness, turns a worrying shade of white. But eventually we reach some sort of plateau, and decide to stop for lunch.

We find ourselves in Santa Lucía, essentially a strip of road in the middle of nowhere, on top of a mountain, but with a surprisingly busy restaurant. It has an open terrace at the back, where we set up camp with our prams and high chairs. The place is run by three white-jacketed brothers: big, squat boisterous men, who move nimbly as ballet dancers, with high-piled plates, becoming ever faster on their feet as the restaurant fills up with locals and tourists. There is an excellent octopus and vinaigrette salad, with large sticks of white asparagus, and aioli to dip. I order a Canarish stew, similar to a Greek stifado: lamb, chickpeas, chorizo, chili, mint, and a rich sauce ideal for mopping up with bread. Ideal, that is, if you have the use of both of your hands, and you are anywhere near the table. Anita and I take it in turns to make laps around the restaurant with Emily, singing 'Row Your Boat' softly to her. One of the brothers, the handsome one, sees me. 'I take two children,' he says (I think he means 'have'), 'I know what it's like.' And he mimes a terrible, robbed-of-sleep yawn with his free hand.

When I return to the table, I notice that the cloud deck, already ominously low, has descended even further. The mountains around us are dissolving slowly into the mist. It's then I remember we're 2,000 metres above sea level. Earlier, we joked about the possibility of a rainstorm: wouldn't like to be stuck up here if that happens!

Then it starts.

A downpour of terrifying force. Great sheets of water sluice from the green tarpaulin roof of the terrace above our heads, into the vines and orange trees below. Emily seems to find it hilarious. She raises her hands to ear-level, and flaps them wildly while laughing. We sit soggily, watching the rain fall for nearly an hour, ordering more beers, and slowly realising we are stranded in what looks like Borneo in monsoon season.

Finally, aware that we could be here all day and all night – perhaps even all week – we ask for *la cuenta*, and make a dash for the car. The brothers wave goodbye with their greasy white towels, and wish us luck.

The drive back down is even more hair-raising than the ascent. I have visions of the brakes failing. The roads are slick and treacherous, and boulders have been loosened. They appear without warning in the middle of the road, like asteroids. But as we inch along the hairpin bends, the rain starts to clear. Suddenly, we see an incredible sight. Far below us, on a plain, is a rainbow. We are high above it, so it appears as a *circular* pool of psychedelic light. God's own lava lamp, smashed open and spilt on a valley floor. We stop for a moment. I take a bad photograph.

Gradually, the roads become straighter, the altitude decreases, the cloud lifts, and the sun makes an appearance. The minutes of suffocating, fist-clenching, feet-pressed-to-the-floor mortal fear become, happily, fewer and fewer. Emily still wails in the back, and Anita still looks pale, but we're down unscathed, and, in the distance, we glimpse the sea, its surface glittering in the sun.

Shortly before the end of our stay, Emily celebrates her first birthday. ('Celebrates' might be the wrong verb.) We make her a breakfast tortilla, with a single candle, which I help to blow out. She cries; we sing. *Happy Birthday!* (Or maybe it should have been 'Unhappy Birthday', the Morrissey song.)

Later that day, as I'm walking Emily through the town in her buggy, the proprietor of a nail bar leaps out of her empty shop and engages us in conversation. She's possibly 50, but looks older, her face smoked to a kipper-ish brown by years of sun and sea-salt. A voluble, gestural woman: prone to theatrical outbursts during our brief exchange. She is bare-footed, and her many bracelets jangle. On one baked forearm is a small, amateurish blue heart tattoo, with a jagged line down the middle: broken. Yet she smiles furiously, showing tiny backward-sloping yellow teeth, her little honey-coloured eyes disappearing into their deep orbits. She wears a white shawl, like a fortune teller.

I'm assailed with questions. When she learns my wife is German, the woman says she speaks a little, and remarks that they make excellent spouses: *Gute köche!* When she sees Emily in the buggy, she almost explodes in rapture.

'Oh, *suess!*'

She rushes to the back of the shop to fetch something, and returns with one of those deeply sinister painted dolls. At least *I* think they're sinister, some people must like them. It has a white crocheted dress, and its hands hold a twisted flamenco pose. Its wig is strawberry blonde, and unpleasantly thick.

The woman kneels down in front of the buggy to make eye contact with Emily, who isn't crying now, but quietly bemused. I make a mental note to spend more time in the town, speaking to eccentric shopkeepers.

'A princess for a Princess!' she says. It's a gift. Does she know it's Emily's birthday? I haven't told her. 'Do you like that I present you with a doll? A Canarish doll?'

She begins to stroke Emily's legs, as if applying sun cream.

'Oh, you're tired! *Müde, ja?* I can see that.'

It might be time to make an exit. I mumble my goodbyes, and move off, only daring to look back once. The woman is waving frantically, bracelets leaping.

'*Tschüss! Tschüss!*'

For the remainder of the holiday, the doll sits silently in a corner of the sofa, shunned, or is moved from high shelf to high shelf. On the last day, I know I can't take the thing home with us. Everyone believes it to be sinister now, not just me. A witch-doll. Even little Billy is wary of it. I go to the back of the villa, and leave it quietly among our bottle mountain, waiting for the van to come.

4

Spider And I

NOVEMBER. WE'VE BEEN back for a while now. The holiday has become a faded memory, something that it might even be possible to laugh about. In ten years' time, perhaps. When we touched down at an autumnal Heathrow, it was as if a switch had been thrown in Emily's brain. She started to smile. By the time we were in the lifts, she was giggling at her shoes. No, Emily, I tried to explain, you've got it the wrong way around: on holiday – happy! Back home – *sad*. We bade farewell to Andrew, Carrie and Billy, promising to have a wine and photo evening soon. They seemed somewhat nervous at the suggestion.

'Darling, shall we listen to the Cluster album?'

These aren't words I ever thought I'd say to my one-year-old daughter, yet this morning, I do. I'm making a start on the new music. So far, I've been immersing myself in the pioneering German avant-rock bands of the early seventies. All of them have great names: Cluster, Amon Düül, Harmonia, Faust, Popol Vuh, *Neu!* ... Cluster is my favourite, a moniker suggestive of vast agglomerations of stars – fitting for 'The Great *Kosmische Musik*' – or the opposite perhaps: tiny molecular structures seen under a microscope. I like to know plenty of background information about a group I'm investigating, so I do some research. Cluster were from Berlin, yet the album I'm listening to, *Sowiesoso*, was recorded in Forst, Lower Saxony, in 1976. (Now *that* would make a great band name. 'I really like some of the early Forst stuff ...') The second pressing of the LP reverses the original back and front images to show the two chief band members, Dieter Moebius and Hans-Joachim Roedelius, standing by bare trees in weak winter sunlight. Behind them, a lake glimmers palely. The photograph has the same grainy, washed-out tones of John Lennon's *Plastic Ono Band* sleeve. I translate some of the track names, using a dubious German-to-English site. *Umleitung*: 'detour'. This is my favourite German word at the moment, along with *Sabberlätzchen*: 'bib'.

But it is the music that grips. It feels utterly modern. It could, as they say, have been recorded yesterday. Soft-focus analogue synths; torpid, pastoral melodies. As the calming sounds fill the living room, Emily stares out of the window at the damp street below, a look of solemn concentration on her face. Then I find a video of Can's exuberant, disco-influenced 'I Want More' on YouTube, and jump around the lounge to it with Emily in my arms. Astonishingly, the song charted: the clip is from *Top of the Pops 2*. Holger Czukay is hunched over a double bass. The young audience appear scandalised by his already greying hair. Guitarist Michael Karoli looks like Lou Reed, the Kevin Keegan Years. 'How on earth did these avant-garde chappies get on *Top of the Pops?*' the strapline commentary reads. 'Democracy is a wonderful thing.' When the song ends I put Emily down on the playmat. She looks happy, and strangely relieved to be back on terra firma.

An episode from the holiday is troubling me. Anita and I are sitting at the little table by the villa's pool, eating a mushroom risotto and ham omelette. We have plenty of aioli, and an abundant supply of the delicious, piquant red sauce we found in the local supermarket. Cervantes beer. Good bread. Emily is napping, and the sun is pleasingly warm on our arms and necks. Everything is agreeable, in other words, but something, we know, is wrong.

Emily.

'She's one, and can't even crawl,' I say, taking a pull on my beer, 'she has no real motor skills to speak of, no sign of any language yet. And the crying ...'

'She's just a late developer, that's all,' says Anita.

True, I know that children hit their milestones at different times – I've read a couple of parenting manuals – but I've been studying little Billy, quietly making comparisons. He can complete entire puzzles; point to his nose or ears when prompted. Emily has a rudimentary grip, but, increasingly, toys reduce her to tears. Andrew and Carrie have given her birthday presents: playthings she can't play with. One is a simple jigsaw, and I watch – filled with envy – as Billy takes over, fitting the pieces into the correct spaces. And emotionally, he just seems more balanced. Yes, boys can tend to be, but Billy is conspicuously unvarying: calm, composed, a little cheeky sometimes, those blue old-man-river eyes taking everything in. His jaw set at all times against Emily's cries of frustration.

'Perhaps that's what it is,' I say. 'She's simply frustrated because she can't really *do* anything yet.'

I push my plate away. The NHS one-year developmental review is due soon, we'll see what answers that yields. But for the first time I experience a stab of fear, somewhere in my lower intestine, that there might actually be something wrong with our daughter's development.

Back in the high-windowed flat, steam issues in great jets from the boiler flue next door. The leaves are almost entirely stripped from the trees now, exposing St Andrew's ugly, chimney-like spire, visible from the kitchen. Emily's crying still preoccupies me. It has improved since Gran Canaria, but can rise without warning from a constant fretful whimper to a roaring, red-faced bellow in seconds. Her anguish seems limitless, emerging from some deep, primitive place. And the doll haunts me: a doll is, after all, an effigy of a child that can't move.

I try to focus on the holiday's happier moments. She loved being held up to paddle in the surf, watching the wave's foam draw back swiftly through her toes, even though she didn't like the island's gritty, dark grey sand. The measured repetition of the sea's motion delighted her. Coming and going, coming and going. But the crying would soon start, and we'd pack our things, leaving Andrew, Carrie, and little Billy playing happily with his bucket and spade.

One night, not long after we return to England, Emily wakes at 3am and cries bitterly for a full hour. This, in itself, isn't unusual, but something is different. Her eyes scan the ceiling of her room in fear, as if it is about to cave in. She seems disorientated, terrified, her expression says: *where am I? What is this strange place?* I've always been aware that she's sensitive to changes in her surroundings, but this disturbs me. Everything is tried: Calpol, rocking, taking her into our bed. In the end, only songs work. Well, one song, 'Row Your Boat', repeated over and over like a mantra.

Row, row, row your boat,
Gently down the stream,
Merrily, merrily, merrily, merrily,
Life is but a dream.

Eventually she settles, but I don't. I lie awake, listening to mother and baby's breathing, haunted by visions of the hire car's brakes failing on that mountain road, and something else, some sort of darkness I cannot fathom.

Morning arrives in an evil fog of exhaustion. I go about the routine like an automaton: boil the kettle, leave it for 25 minutes, clean the small stainless-steel flask, fill it for Emily's milk. Then I go into her room to check on her. When I draw the orange curtains, she smiles with delight. She seems to have made a full recovery, the terrors of the night forgotten. A moment later, Anita appears beside me. 'What's my name again?' she says, weariness in her big grey eyes. Then, holding Emily up so she can stand and grip the bars of the cot with both hands: 'Won't it be great when we find her in the morning, doing this on her own?'

I agree, but in my secret heart I fear that day might be a long time in the future.

*

I'm applying myself to the search for new music, but it's already becoming a chore. And making a list of Emily's discoveries also feels like a task – not because there are so many, but because there are so few.

I can't face any of the choppy, beardy bands yet, so I look for some pop. I stumble upon a Taylor Swift video, 'Blank Space', on YouTube. Swift is hardly new, but I click on 'play' all the same. She wears a different outfit every four seconds. It has 1,117,193, 903 views. I look at the figure again. That's over a billion, isn't it? This sort of highly machined pop leaves me feeling skittery, as if I've just drunk a Starbucks Grande latte. Or two. I feel like I need to have a lie-down. But she's clearly a good pop star, striding confidently through a landscape of post-postmodern visual signifiers, even parodying Lady Gaga at one point.

Then I discover Julia Holter. I've been saving her, actually, knowing with awful music-snob clarity that she'll be right up my street. Domino records; the sleeve photograph that recalls PJ Harvey, Laura Nyro, or *Horses*-era Patti Smith; the breathless reviews that reference 17th-century madrigals and French impressionist classical music, already skim-read. The songs on her album, *Have You in My Wilderness*, are intimate, lucid, mysterious. Moments of silence give way to unexpected

Jimmy Webb chord shifts. Shonky saxophone breaks emerge from nowhere. And above this, Holter's voice: assured, supple, beguiling. She's brilliant.

But she's not Kate Bush.

I decide not to play any of Holter's stuff to Emily. Only the original, and best, for my daughter.

*

'Can she say "Mummy" or "Daddy", or any vocalism containing a consonant followed by a vowel?' asks the woman.

It is the day of the one-year developmental review, and the woman is a health visitor, sitting on the playmat in our lounge with Emily and Anita. She's keen to project a brisk, professional manner, yet seems approachable and kind, too. I'm sitting slumped and suffering with flu at the dining table. There is a lengthy questionnaire to be completed.

'No,' I reply.

'Can she hold anything, such as a pencil?'

'No. I mean, yes. A spoon held lightly in her fist. But not a pinch grip.'

'Does she point at an object she wants?'

'No.'

'Can she crawl, bum-slide, or walk?'

'No.'

'Can she stand up unassisted?'

'No.'

Finally, I say, 'Are you concerned about any of this?'

The woman's composure slips for a brief moment. She looks into the middle distance, like an actor trying to remember a line.

'I'm not really here to have *concerns*, as such,' she says, smiling, 'just to get answers to some questions.'

There is a palpable climate of anxiety in the room, coming from the worried parents. (All right, from me. Anita is playing naturally with Emily, radiating a stoic-ism that I can only admire.)

I try pressing the health visitor again. She admits that Emily has indeed scored very low. On the questionnaire, the 'no's' are ominous black circles. On the last page is a sort of graph, or table, with a cluster of them on the left, gradually merging with grey 'don't knows' in the middle, then white 'yes's' on the right. She indicates that, when the results are compiled and passed on to the paediatrician's monthly meeting for assessment – which she will push for personally – Emily is more than likely going to be in the black.

The meeting over, I make some brief notes on the health visitor's activity suggestions, then return to my sickbed. It's a blowy, darkening November afternoon, the yellow plane trees in the back garden stretching themselves into odd shapes. Anita appears, sits on the edge of the bed. A shadow seems to pass over her face, her eyes widen, cheeks redden, and tears come.

'She mentioned "play therapy",' she says, weeping gently. 'That's what the children with learning difficulties have to do at my school.'

'What, like special needs?' I ask, fear in my voice.

'Yes, sometimes.'

Wild autumn is here. Thin rain. Mean wind. Unruly trees. Leaf litter everywhere. The windows of the flat, long overdue a clean, are misted. I've been subdued after the previous day's meeting, trying to formulate a plan of action. The health visitor suggested we try assisted walking. Now, with the light slipping away again at 4pm, I can hear Emily being put through her paces with Anita in the next room.

'Good, Emily! Bravo!'

Then the sound of our daughter's throaty growl of effort as she takes a few faltering, facilitated steps. The health visitor also suggested repeating words, to promote speech. I will say 'Mummy' (or '*Mama*', the preferred German form of 'Mummy') and 'Daddy' to her until she's sick of them. In fact, I will do it in the form of drumming, a paradiddle on my thighs (a pattern of four even strokes, played in the order 'left right, left right', similar to the rhythm of Led Zeppelin's 'Boogie With Stu'). According to the drummers I know who also teach, this is how you actually learn a paradiddle.

Mum-my, Dad-dy,
Mum-my, Dad-dy…

Repeated again and again, becoming ever faster.

The project fills me with fresh hope. Yet when I observe Emily attempting to eat her Weetabix with the spoon held so lightly, so precariously in her fist – which she drops instantly after a mouthful – I'm reminded of a disabled boy I knew when I was younger. I try to edge the thought to the back of my mind.

My father and his partner, Joan, come over to Surbiton one Sunday for lunch. They are both in their late seventies. I'm slightly nervous; I still don't know how much to tell them. A baby is such a joy that to reveal anything might be wrong could cause alarm, embarrassment, a discordant scene. When he phones me from the station, I stumble over my words.

But once I've collected them, and the first glass of red is poured, I relax somewhat. Anita's *Sauerbraten* – a German beef stew served with dumplings and a deliquescent cream and leak sauce – is much-praised. However, before long, the inevitable subject of Emily's 'delay' is raised. When I describe her lack of progress and odd behaviours, Joan looks concerned. She has two grown-up sons from a previous marriage, one of them – Richard – the disabled boy Emily briefly reminded me of. (Or 'mentally handicapped', as she says, the term of choice from the 1970s.)

Richard is now in his late forties, slightly older than me, and living in full-time residential care. When he was a baby, his parents didn't suspect anything was untoward until he was a year and a half. 'He just sat there smiling, doing nothing,' says Joan. My chest constricts. This is what Emily does, more or less. What if …? What if her oxygen was compromised at birth, or something? I'd always believed that this was the reason for Richard's disability, but when I mention it, Joan says no, the cause was never established. So how had I got that in my head? I think back to Richard as an adolescent: a ball of conflicting energies like a normal teenager, but with the 'mental age of a two-year-old' (the phrase that was used then). I remember the ripe smell from his trousers as he soiled himself, his rapid hand movements, his hoarse cries of delight or confusion. He was epileptic, too, and I once witnessed him suffer a *grand mal* seizure in front of me. In truth, I was scared of him. But what I recall most is the parents' touching devotion. They would visit Richard at his special care home every day. This moved me, even as a boy.

Joan, sitting next to me, turns and places a hand on mine.

'I know the worry you're going through, my darling.'

Hang on.

What the HELL are you talking about? How dare you equate Emily with Richard?

I don't say this.

Instead, I mumble the party line, that Emily is just a 'late bloomer', which I now desperately want to believe myself. I pour myself another large glass of red, and pick at the cold *Sauerbraten* in silence as the conversation drifts to other matters.

A few days later, I take Emily to the Health Centre. (Yet another ear infection. 'Welcome to the nursery years,' said Dr Daly, on our last visit.) All the way, brown leaf-mulch, slippery as wallpaper paste, sticks to the pram's wheels. A weak afternoon sunset shows pink behind the chimney pots. Skeins of Canadian geese pass high overhead, in V formation – the exodus south to the warm countries has begun; a melancholy annual sight in Surbiton. More and more glide above, wave after wave, in long processions, like bombers.

I'm in a deep depression after my father's visit, brooding on my daughter's delayed development. I have to dislodge these thoughts somehow. She will be perfectly all right.

Won't she?

I stare at Emily's tiny, plump hands on the roll bar of the pram. When I sing 'The Wheels On The Bus', she flaps them like birds' wings, something she does quite a lot – and odd, 'vogue-ing' movements with her fingers; her 'Shirley Bassey shapes' as I call them. I crane my neck over the pram's hood to see her face: she's smiling, at least.

After the appointment, a prescription for antibiotics and infant ibuprofen in hand, I drop into the supermarket. At the checkout, a mum in front of us says to her toddler:

'Do you want to put the goodies on the belt?'

'Yes, Mummy,' replies the little boy, who can only be six months older than Emily.

I feel a surge of painful emotion. I want to be able to ask my daughter that question, to hear her say, 'Yes, Daddy'.

When we return to the flat, I lay Emily down for her nap, and put an old record on. Brian Eno's 'Spider And I', from *Before and After Science*. But quietly, so I won't wake her. Then I go into the main bedroom, and lie down on top of the bed. The song floats in like a ghost from the lounge. On the line about sleeping in the morning, great racking sobs come up from nowhere. Spasms that I can't control. My eyes are so completely full of tears I can't see. Eventually, it subsides, but the violence of the episode frightens me. I draw a breath deep into my lungs, then exhale.

Breathe. Breathe. Breathe.

5

Wish You Were Here

'ARE EITHER OF you perfectionists?'

We are in our local gastro pub with an NCT couple we like but don't know very well. The husband, Tim, a doctor – tall, with sandy hair – has just asked me a direct question. He is smiling shyly.

Anita and I turn to each other. There is an opportunity for a joke here, a piece of marital badinage, but it's a serious question he's asking.

'Only my wife,' I say, provocatively.

It gets a laugh, but the point he's making is: maybe Emily has inherited this. Tim quickly admits to being a perfectionist himself, in case he's been too forward. It's possible, he says, that her intelligence is ahead of her motor skills, hence the frustration with toys. This is the best possible scenario, I say, although perhaps it's just what a worried father wants to hear. Recently, in his company, I've found myself asking Tim anxious questions about Emily's development. I know it's impertinent to do this with an off-duty medical professional, but I've heard he makes exceptions with some of the other NCT parents.

Cassandra, Tim's wife, is standing next to us with their daughter, little Tia, on her hip. I watch Tia put a small piece of bread roll in her mouth. Something about the movement of the wrist, the smooth turn, has a sophistication that is completely absent in Emily's motor skills-set. But I'm comparing again.

Tim, casting around for any advice he can give, says that when Tia was late to crawl he took her outside to the garden, where there was soil and grass. For some reason this was the trigger. She began crawling, and now she can walk.

Do we need to find a trigger?

Christmas is six weeks away. In the centre of town, a crane lowers the stock of a Norwegian spruce tree into a cavity in a roundabout. In the supermarkets, couples with children drop tubes of wrapping paper and boxes of Belgian chocolates into their trolleys. In the pubs, festive songs are beginning to be heard on sound systems, an early trickle of tinsel and whisky. And above Surbiton: cardboard skies, a uniform grey like the inside of a cereal box. Cold November rain, as Axl Rose once sang, strafes the rooftops. A single maple leaf, brown and flimsy, pirouettes in the air. I hold Emily up to the window to watch it. We are in the lounge, as usual, just the two of us. The Beatles' 'Blackbird' is playing on the stereo. The lines about broken wings and learning to fly, waiting for freedom, feel terribly apt.

A memory of a recent conversation with Anita, in the same room, returns: I decided to share my fear that Emily was disabled. She paused to consider this, but I don't think she believed it.

'Everyone is telling us how much Emily is progressing,' I said, 'and, oh, so- and-so couldn't walk until they were 16 months. But that just makes it worse, somehow. I know they mean well but ... I can't see it. Perhaps I'm just too close to it all.'

A sharp exchange followed.

'I'm just concerned about our daughter,' I said, 'but I'm trying to get on with it. Normal life, that is.'

'You've only smiled twice in a week.'

'It was once.'

Back in the present, the memory of my facetious remark still stinging, I reflect that Anita has found her optimism since her tears in the bedroom. She seems to be handling the situation better than me. I need to be strong for my daughter, too. I hold Emily up higher so she can see the green birds fleeing the copper beech tree, one by one. Then I sit her on my knee and drum along to Sister Sledge's 'We Are Family'. The paradiddle.

Mum-my, Dad-dy. Mum-my, Dad-dy ...

*

A text from a friend wakes me in the morning: 'All those poor people in Paris.' What has happened? I open Twitter. There's been another terrorist atrocity, maybe 200 dead. Climbing out of bed, I realise it probably won't be long until London is targeted again.

I have an intimation that it's going to be a strange day. At noon, the NCT group's first-birthday-party-for-all-the-babies is being held at a church hall in Long Ditton. We pack our old Renault Clio in an angry rainstorm – a lemon cake, a tightly cling-filmed bowl of salad, a six-pack of Beck's, a red Bobby Car; presents and cards for the other children. On the way there, Emily wails unstoppably in the back, strapped into her Maxi-Cosi car seat. We park, and stumble through the dripping graveyard with our burden of gifts and toys. The headstones and the trees seem especially slick and vivid, glistening in the meagre light. Water droplets collect under the wingtips of an imposing carved angel. It strikes me that the venue is grimly appropriate for such a sombre day.

As we push through the double doors to the capacious hall, a tumult of voices greets us. Everyone from the group is here – seven sets of parents and their children. Our socio-economic profile is slightly different, to say the least, from the other mums and dads. They are mostly doctors, lawyers, accountants. Anita is a part-time primary school teacher; I'm a writer who plays guitar in jazz and blues dives. We borrowed the 250 quid to join. I was ready for the group to consist of golfers and wankers, but, annoyingly, everyone is perfectly nice. They're all good people.

Keeping an eye on Emily, who is sitting with the other children on a giant playmat, I sip champagne from a paper cup, and pick at food from a plate. Quiche, Coronation chicken; generously large homemade sausage rolls. I talk to Tim about the Paris massacre, and Emily, of course. So far, he's the only one we've confided in about her delay.

There is an additional motive for my attendance today. I want to scrutinise the other children, measure their level of development against Emily's. They are all mobile in some form or other, and engage with toys, the fine motor skills of their fingers enabling them to explore, pick up objects, release them. The Bobby Car is commandeered and pitted against a First Steps Baby Walker in a race. But Emily is soon in tears, flapping her hands in frustration. After several attempts to help her play with the others, I realise she's exhausted, and find a corner of the hall to place her in a makeshift bed. My warm winter coat and Anita's voluminous orange cardigan suffice. This isolation, I realise, symbolises our daughter's outsider status, but I don't mention it to Anita, who is chatting happily to the other parents. I just feel an overwhelming sadness that Emily can't join in with her playmates. But she seems to like her cosy new crib, looking up at me, grinning, and I pull funny faces to make her laugh.

It's soon past four o'clock – we must be out by five. There is a hasty group photograph in front of a large 'One' at the back of the hall. A milestone: one whole year of life. After the clear-up, we struggle in the dark through the still-dripping graveyard, laden down with coats and bags and the Bobby Car, and make our way to the Renault.

It's only later, in the flat, over a glass of wine, that I take a look at a homemade book one of the NCT mothers has had printed for each of the parents. It contains photographs of all the children throughout their first year. On the back cover is a collage of the babies' names, and random words made from fridge magnets. I stop dead. It begins:

Only Emily
Try Tomorrow
About Hope

*

Each morning, instead of pursuing the new music project, I carry out a series of balance and movement exercises with my daughter. First, I stand her up by the lounge window so she can grip the low sill, which is roughly shoulder height for her. Then, with one hand for extra support at the small of her back, I use my other hand to plant her feet wider, enabling better equilibrium. She stands quietly, looking down at the street below. I take off her socks so her feet have more traction, and her odd toes splay out like a monkey's. I'm acutely aware she will eventually collapse sideways or backwards if I remove my steadying hand. Then we 'walk': me holding her under her arms, circumnavigating the playmat. Ten, 20, 30, 40 paces. Each time, her right foot extends in one great lunging step. She barks with effort – *Ah!* – but I can see she's excited, focused, happy. Proud. We rest, then start again from a sitting position. She can now grip both my index fingers and lift herself to stand.

Next we raid the toy box. Some of them definitely 'do' too much. I can see her becoming frustrated and angry at the profusion of flashing lights, sped-up voices, blaring song fragments. She is far calmer playing with the string on my fleece, or combing my hair with her fingers, or exploring the texture of the keypad on an old cordless phone. Sitting down, engaging with actual playthings designed for toddlers is more problematic. She grabs a plastic hoop, but doesn't seem to know what to do with it, except bash it repetitively on the floor. Almost always, this is when the crying starts. Then she throws the hoop down – it spins off until it is far away. And because she cannot crawl over to retrieve it, her frustration is doubled. After this, she picks up the red telephone that belongs to the Baby Walker with both hands. This is encouraging, but then she starts smashing it against the main body of the toy, like Robert De Niro in the phone-box scene from *Goodfellas*. What's more, it ends up covered in spit. She's going through a dribbling phase – teething, we think – which is enchanting, of course.

At the NCT party, Tim asked if Emily was responsive to music. She is, I said. He suggested buying her a keyboard, or a drum. Apart from the fact she doesn't have the fine motor skills yet, I had to admit the idea of a drum scared me slightly. Our downstairs neighbours, Anna and Roberto, a friendly Italian couple with two young children, recently had a mini drum kit delivered. We haven't heard it in use. Yet.

In the days that follow, I opt for some quieter pleasures: Bill Evans' *Paris Concert* on CD. Emily is bewitched. Is it the flurries of piano notes that rise up seemingly from nowhere? The sinuous snap of Marc Johnson's double bass? The ghostly applause between songs, like autumn leaves crunching far away? It's hard to tell, but her response is marked. One morning, I put on Bach's *St Matthew Passion* while I feed her Weetabix, mashed banana and strawberries. She looks up thoughtfully, following the four-part chorale – heavenly voices that appear to float out eerily from the mezzanine above us.

Later, I take the acoustic guitar out of its case and play her a song – a shaky rendition of Pink Floyd's 'Wish You Were Here', hoping to add it to Emily's setlist. She sits utterly spellbound – the best audience I've ever had. She is wide-eyed with astonishment at what she is hearing and seeing. The line about the two lost souls in the fishbowl, that could be us, I think, during the long afternoons when I have to devise new ways to entertain her. Prospero and Miranda, marooned on the island. Donald and Kate on the hill – *It's you and me, Daddy*. The Gruffalo and the Gruffalo's child … Then I have an idea. I dig out the small, red, charity-shop tambourine from the depths of the toy box, and put on disc two of the Beatles' *White Album*. She's thrilled with this new plaything, and doesn't discard it immediately, instead, bashing crudely away with both hands to 'Birthday', 'Everybody's Got Something To Hide Except Me And My Monkey', 'Helter Skelter'. On the gentler tracks, the beautiful, hymn-like 'Mother Nature's Son', the strange, shadow-filled 'Long, Long, Long', I sing along, ghosting the melody. Then I dance her around to 'Honey Pie', doing McCartney's flapper voice, the one he used to impress his father. Her eyes are alight.

It feels like winter now, as I push Emily in the buggy to the doctors, fingers of pink and grey cloud showing in an icy blue sky. The last of the migrating geese, small dark arrowheads, passing silently overhead.

In the consulting room, Emily sits on my knee in her red snowsuit, giggling whenever Dr Daly hits the clacking keys of her old NHS computer. Even though we're here for advice about an ear infection, I restate my worries over Emily's lack of movement, her difficulty with toys. I say we're still waiting to hear from the hospital about a paediatrician's appointment. Did the health visitor, who promised to make the referral herself, forget? Dr Daly doesn't know. Privately, I vow never to be caught out like this again, to always make the call myself.

Valuable time has been lost, and I'm desperate for some answers.

Dr Daly seems embarrassed, and apologises profusely. Call the paediatric secretary, she says, and if you have no luck, leave a message here and she will push from this end. In the meantime, she'll try to have Emily fast-tracked to see a physiotherapist at somewhere called Harefield House. It's these small acts of kindness, knowing that someone other than me and Anita is concerned about Emily's progress, that are moving. I don't know if she's aware of what it means to me. I thank her three times.

Walking back, I reflect on the parlous money situation. Anita and I are just working, working, working to pay the bills, trapped in an apparently endless round of toil. We'll just about survive Christmas, if we're lucky. A gift amnesty has been declared; holidays cancelled or postponed. (The trip to Gran Canaria was ruinous.) On Saturday, Anita admitted she hasn't been this poor since she was a student. I feel a terrible burden upon me, a duty to support my family – I'm meant to be able to 'provide'. The rent will go up next year, travel costs will inevitably rise … What's more, there is much concern in London now about a Paris-style 'mass casualty' terrorist attack. Shootings, or a bomb. Perhaps we should move? There must be a better place, a cheaper place. We've been talking idly about this; leaving for Germany to be nearer Anita's parents. And Emily, with all her difficulties, would have a paediatrician there (extraordinarily, all doctors who treat children in Germany are paediatricians, not just general practitioners). Yes, she would probably be better off over there.

*

'So what's wrong with her?' asks the sullen voice at the other end of the telephone.

I've finally got through to the paediatric secretary, and am trying to stay calm, although I'm feeling rage. I'm aware that the NHS is desperately overstretched – and any attack on them feels like an attack on my mother, who worked as a nurse for 40 years – but they have no record of a referral, and I'm having to go back to the start, reiterating all of Emily's symptoms.

'Well, she's 13 months old and can't do anything, not even crawl,' I reply.

'Oh. OK. Can you fax the developmental review over?'

Fax? Is it 1995?

I keep cool, and agree to fax it, if that is their preferred method of communication. Then I phone the surgery and leave a message for Dr Daly to make a fresh referral, just in case.

A late winter's afternoon in the flat. Anita is putting up the Christmas decorations. Snowflake lights trail across the lounge window, and bright red tinsel garlands the ladder to the mezzanine. Carols play on the stereo. I feel hopeful. Emily's legs are becoming stronger, her steps more evenly balanced. Each time she completes an assisted lap of the playmat – a look of focus and happy determination on her face – we cheer and give applause. I ruffle her unruly mop of blonde hair. 'Where are you going, Bear?' I ask. She grins with delight, and I notice her eyes are changing colour, slowly, surely, to match her mother's. The same complex range of greys, flecked with gold.

Mid-December. I am in the lounge with Emily. We stare out of the window at brutalist skies, murderous ravens; the last leaves on the copper beech shivering helplessly in the wind. She is completely absorbed, following blackbirds that soar up to a maple tree; or crows, gulls and pigeons that wheel overhead, riding the currents, treading air, then dropping swiftly out of the sky. I'm certain she could stand here all day, gripping the window sill until her legs give out. Her calm, sentient gaze ... She looks so beautiful in profile that I want to take a photograph, but my phone has reached maximum memory capacity – mostly due to shots of her – and, anyway, the immovable ridge of green snot on her left nostril would perhaps preclude it from being among my favourites.

I've noticed something else lately. The smallest things make her laugh. This is better than the crying, but it puzzles me somewhat. She'll catch herself in the mirrored wardrobe doors and start giggling. Or Anita will 'snap' some damp washing like a bullfighter, and there will be gusts of laughter. Odd things amuse her. Unfunny stuff. Slapstick. *Goodies*-type sketches. Sketches *The Goodies* would have rejected. I accidentally roll a biro off the dining table: hysterics.

A letter from Harefield House arrives. I tear it open, standing in the common area downstairs by the mail pigeonholes. It's the physiotherapist's referral. Outcome: 'accepted'. A wave of elation sweeps over me, then I notice the address: *Harefield House. Integrated service for children with disabilities.* I feel as if I've been winded, knocked off a horse. I put the letter down.

Then I sit on the first step, and stare at the Victorian fanlight above the front door.

So Emily *is disabled.*

Later, with our daughter asleep in her room, silently watching TV on the sofa in the darkened lounge, Anita suddenly asks: 'What do you feel in your gut? Is she special needs?'

I glance at her. My wife is staring straight ahead. I notice the television light reflected in her right eye, glistening.

And still we wait for Emily to move. All the measures we planned to implement months ago have faltered: setting plants on high shelves in case she eats the soil; installing batteries instead of power cords for electrical appliances; laying down new rugs to prevent her gashing herself on exposed nails. She shows no sign of crawling or walking unassisted. If there is a trigger, I can't think of one. Furthermore, Anita receives a continual bombardment of WhatsApp updates from the other NCT mums, which only serve to accentuate our daughter's lack of progress. All *their* children are mobile, powering ahead.

Today is sunlit and glittering, a pure, sharp December day. On the way back from nursery, Emily shouts with Blake-ean joy. Yet I just can't imagine her with movement or speech. *This is her, now*, I think to myself.

*

'Er, this is the library.'

The woman behind the reception desk looks worried. A crazy man is standing before her with a small child over his shoulder, dripping from a rainstorm. The man is me. It is the day of the paediatrician's appointment – finally, we've been granted one – and we're late. Anita is driving around in the rain somewhere, looking for a parking space in the one-way, double-yellow-line hell of Kingston town centre. And I'm in the wrong part of a many-floored concrete building where the clinic is supposed to be.

'A map on the letter would've helped,' I mumble, knowing it's not her fault, or problem. But I'm consumed by a terrible urgency, as I know the clinic will send us away if we're more than ten minutes late – and it's taken months to gain this appointment.

The woman offers me directions, and within moments the correct receptionist is asking me to take a seat in a packed, chapel-quiet waiting room. With panic, I realise I don't have a dummy, as I leapt out of the Renault without the baby bag. But mercifully, for once, Emily sits in silence on my knee, gazing benevolently at the person next to her.

A diminutive nurse calls us, and Emily's weight and height are measured in a chilly, featureless room. Then we are sent back to the waiting area. Anita arrives, and before long we are summoned to see the senior consultant paediatrician, Dr McNally. His hooded eyes extend a hint of a smile as he welcomes us into his office, a space devoid of the expected toys or animal wall stickers. He is bald on top, but with plentiful red hair at the sides, and wears a wide-collared shirt under a blue cord blazer. Slacks, black loafers, gold watch. It's a quietly dandy-ish look, and slightly incongruous, given the gravity of his role. A cravat wouldn't look out of place, cresting above the open neck of the shirt.

We pour out everything we can about our daughter's history, her development, or lack of it. The troubled birth, the colic, the crying, the laughing, the problems with mobility, the paucity of motor skills – Anita and I confirming or contradicting each other's observations. It's a shambolic performance, but the basic backstory is established.

During this, Emily is calm, and Anita sporadically walks her around the consulting office. McNally listens attentively, then asks for our daughter to be stripped down to her nappy. This done, he kneels in front of her to conduct a brief examination. It has the feel of a nativity scene, the genuflecting wise man before the holy infant ... The room falls silent for the first time since the meeting began. He shines a small torch in her eyes, taps her kneecaps with a tiny wooden mallet, checks her lymph glands. He's gentle with her. Finally, he tries to interest her in one of the few toys from a cardboard box on a shelf, but Emily doesn't interact; instead, she pulls away, summoned by something that has caught her attention in a corner.

The paediatrician returns to his chair, and begins to make copious, illegible notes. I attempt to read them furtively but they may as well be hieroglyphics. The room fills with our voices once more, and I'm halfway through another poorly-described account of one of Emily's perplexing behaviours, when Dr McNally lays his gold pen on the desk, looks directly at the two anxious, bewildered people he has in his office, and speaks:

'I'm sorry to say this, but there is a problem.'

6

The Fog

THE ROOM IS very still. Ice flows down my spine.

'There is a delay in her motor skills, social communication and interaction, and her willingness to explore. All these things can get better. But I don't want to say everything is all right.'

Dr McNally pauses, then says: 'Are you OK? Do you need a tissue?'

'Sorry?' I say.

I turn to Anita, and realise he's addressing her. I notice that her left wrist is wet. She's been crying, and tears have dropped down. He pulls out a Kleenex from a square box on his desk, leans over, hands it to her.

McNally continues in a steady, neutral tone. Emily will need a series of investigations. A blood test to check for enzymes; she may have low muscle tone, hypotonia. An X-ray to rule out a misaligned pelvis. An Electroencephalography (EEG) to detect electrical activity – epilepsy or seizures – in the brain. A thyroid function test. A hearing assessment. A genetic assessment. I interject with nervous questions, to which he gives cautious, measured answers. When I ask if he thinks her problems might be related to the difficult birth, he says, no, they're more likely to be genetic in origin.

Then he has a series of questions for us. At one point he queries if we're related. Cousins.

'I have to ask,' he says.

Finally, he proposes the main investigation. An MRI brain scan to determine whether Emily's problems are neurological, if there are any underlying conditions.

'This would require a general anaesthetic, at St Thomas's hospital.'

We shift uncomfortably in our seats. But Emily is so little, she's only one. Aren't there risks involved at that age? I'm not keen, I say. I glance at Anita; she nods in agreement. McNally confirms that there are indeed risks, but suggests we give it serious thought. In any event, we need to come back in three to six months for a follow-up appointment.

The meeting is concluding. I summon my courage and ask: 'On a scale of one to ten, how concerned should we be?' (I'm unable to stop my voice cracking on 'concerned'.)

He pauses, then fixes me with those hooded eyes in which I can read nothing, and replies: 'Five.'

In the cramped box of the lift, Anita's expression is composed, steely. She asks me how I feel about what we've just heard. I don't know how I feel, I say. I'm in shock. Nothing has registered yet.

We find the Renault, strap Emily into her seat, then climb silently in ourselves, Anita in the front, me in the back. As we speed away, our eyes meet in the rear-view mirror.

'I just hope it's physical, not neurological,' says Anita. 'If she's got special needs, we've got a mountain ahead of us.'

*

That night I have a dream – a dream I often used to have as a child. I'm in the sea, treading water, a long way from the shoreline. It's night, and I'm wearing pyjamas; I feel them swell and ride up my calves as I pedal my feet. I'm very cold. My head is barely above the foaming greenish surface, and with tiresome regularity I need to spit out a stream of brine through my teeth. The water is deep, immensely deep; I have a vivid sense that there is nothing underneath me but mile upon mile of ocean; black, invisible depths. It engenders a paradoxical feeling of vertigo – I'm at ground zero, sea level, yet as high as an aeroplane. The vast, torn sky above me somehow confirms this. It is a feeling – and this fascinates me – of being held in a shifting embrace, yet with nothing below but a void; a fly trapped in the meniscus on a glass of water. What's more, being so far out is radically different to the safe coastal areas in which I'm used to swimming as a boy. Here the noise is tremendous. The waves flex and turn with enormous power; I fall and rise as if on a fairground ride, and in one decisive movement can be displaced ten metres to my left or right.

And then, slowly, an apprehension dawns, a cold feeling of dread: if my strength fails, the mouthfuls of saltwater will become hard as rock in my throat, and then in my chest, and I will be drawn choking down towards the abyss.

I wake early, the nightmare still fresh; my mind boiling with fears, outcomes.

A mountain ahead of us.

I throw off the bedclothes, and head for the kitchen. Minute details from the meeting with the paediatrician keep returning – a comment here, a look there. I have to remember them, set them down; they could be significant.

He seemed sure that Emily's problems weren't associated with the birth. But what if something *had* gone wrong? The pregnancy had been uneventful: no falls, no illnesses, no scares. The birth, however, had been anything but. What if our daughter's oxygen had been compromised? What if brain damage had been caused, right then – at that very moment?

*

'She just looks so alert and normal, I can't believe there's anything wrong with her.'

This is Anita, over dinner. We're in the lounge, candles lit, wine in a carafe on the table between us. Her eyes blaze and glitter in the semi-dark. It's four days since the appointment with the paediatrician.

I pick up my glass, and consider this statement. Part of me agrees. Emily doesn't look like a brain-damaged child, and she's just so happy – most of the time.

'You know,' I say, taking a large slug of red, 'I think I was expecting to go into that meeting and the doctor say, she's perfectly all right, you were worrying for nothing.'

We discuss whether to go ahead with the brain scan. Anita has been speaking to some of her closer NCT friends. Apparently, a little girl known to one of the mums went through an MRI under general anaesthetic, only for it to be found her brain was completely normal. So why take the risk?

We agree to wait for the results of the physical tests first.

I come away from the discussion feeling low and drained. I hate the fact that some of the NCT group know that Emily needs a brain scan; that they might feel sorry for us. Yet I have to concede it's useful to share what's happening, in case someone has some information.

Later that evening, at my regular gig in Covent Garden, I confide in two fellow musicians – both fathers – about Emily's issues, hoping to hear that maybe one of their daughters had also been a late developer. I wish I hadn't. One replies: 'She had language early, although she wasn't conjugating French verbs or anything.' We all laugh. But when I start talking about paediatrician appointments and brain scans he becomes uncomfortable, stares into his pint. The other guy, too. So we're on our own then, Anita and I. What I witnessed was the natural recoil of the healthy from the sick.

But *is* Emily sick?

Carluccio's, Kingston. Five days before Christmas. We're here for a rare treat, a late brunch: eggs Florentine, and a children's portion of ravioli for Emily. I watch a young couple nearby, eating lunch with their toddler. 'Olives!' I hear the little girl say, and feel a stab of … what? Longing?

When will Emily say 'Olives'?

After she's finished her food, I walk her around the restaurant.

We pass the table with the couple, and the mother asks how old she is. 'Fifteen months,' I reply. Both parents beam at Emily when they see her broad smile.

When the crying starts, I steer her to the enormous glass frontage that affords a view of a square, and beyond that, the river. I sing 'White Christmas' for her. Outside, in freezing winter weather, ragged pigeons scrabble and strut, and soon Emily is laughing, unable to believe their antics.

We return to our table – a riot of torn, stained napkins, baby snacks, and toys. I clear up as best I can, pay the bill, and leave the largest tip I can afford.

We walk back along Queens Promenade, the river path. The Thames is dotted with geese and rowers, its waters a drab, bark-brown. A strong wind stipples the surface, purling it, and underneath, the current looks powerful, fast-moving. The effect is chaotic: the river is, literally, all over the place. I realise I've always lived near to a river – when I was a boy, it was Hitchin's peculiarly named the *Hiz*.

I push the buggy, while Anita trots ahead, pretending to be a horse for Emily. The red bobble on her hat is leaping up and down. I can hear giggling from the buggy. Soon, I'm chuckling, too. Seize these moments of joy, I tell myself. Recognise their brevity. Never forget them.

A memory returns: a February morning, almost two years ago. Anita walking into the bedroom with a pregnancy test, an unequivocal blue line showing in the small oval window. Oh, how we whooped and leapt with joy! Married for only a few brief months, our attempts to conceive seemed to have worked first time. I was immediately aware of a curious hierarchy of emotions: guilt at our luck when several couples we knew were in the throes of IVF, then a sort of schoolboy pride at having passed on my genes, then apprehensiveness about whether I was equal to the job of being a father. And then a deeper fear … conditions, syndromes, abnormalities.

I did an odd thing. When Anita went to the bathroom to conduct a second test, I made my way to the lounge window, knelt down before the brittle cross on top of St Mark's church, and said a brief, silent prayer:

Please God, don't let the kid have anything wrong with it.

Then I rose swiftly to my feet.

Later, we walked by the river in icy rain and fierce winds, a day not unlike the present one. Back then, however, the Thames was flooding; the water had risen as far as the grass verge where the geese feed. Further ahead, towards the bridge, it looked wild, treacherous. But we were excited at the news, and could talk of nothing else. My prayer from earlier embarrassed me. It seemed, even by my own overly anxious standards, unwarranted, overblown. I hadn't had any religious compunctions since I was a teenager. I kept it to myself.

The low winter sun was huge behind us. We passed the benches with their sad, gentle inscriptions. *A brilliant dad … A favourite walk … In loving memory of … Always with us … He loved the river.* Some were carved directly into the wood, others engraved on burnished plaques, like the nameplates on grand houses. I looked up at the poplars, their peaks striving into the raw blue sky. My heart was full.

I was going to be a dad.

Back in the present, the red bobble still leaping, Emily still laughing, we make our way slowly home. I resolve to take each new development as it comes, not to reach for any conclusions. Let's just see what the following weeks bring.

Twenty-fourth of December. In Surbiton, everyone is work-weary, Christmas-ready. Overheard phone conversations proceed like this: '… Yeah, then I've got to do all my wrapping, and write all my cards.' Every other 4x4 has antlers pinned to the roof. Every other person seems to be wearing a Santa hat. All texts end with 'Merry Xmas'. No one has their mind on anything else, let alone the last dregs of work.

Anita and Emily have already left for her parents in Germany, while I stay in London for my pre-Christmas gigs. Today, I take a cab to Heathrow to join them. I miss my daughter, and have been thinking about a strange episode of *Peppa Pig* we watched together last week. The family drove up into the mountains, got caught in a rainstorm, then saw a rainbow …

The yearning ninths of Wham!'s 'Last Christmas' ring through the airport. I hit the bar, then make my way rapidly to the gate, the plane already boarding. Before long we're up in the air. Soon the jewel case of Frankfurt is laid out to our right. And soon, speeding down the black *autobahn* in my father-in-law's Audi, brooding, invisible forests flash past. Road signs with exciting names loom out of the darkness: *Sprendlingen, Erzhausen, Egelsbach* …

The lights of the town appear, Christmassy and welcoming.

I can't wait to see Emily.

The Fog

Twenty-fifth of December. Morning. I carry my daughter to the living-room window, and we watch the sun crest a belt of silver birch on a low hill in the distance. Mist rises between them, like smoke from extinguished fires – 'the foxes are brewing coffee', as the Germans say. The light glitters on Emily's eyelashes, and gleams on the thick green lanes of snot running from her dainty, retroussé nose.

It's just us in the room.

My in-laws' lounge has a low, wooden, alpine-style ceiling, with a binary light above the dining table, suspended on a metal chain. Two comforting, competing grandfather clocks tick. Everywhere, candles are lit: green, red, gold, their flames reflected in the silverware and pewter kept in glass cabinets. Miniature *Weihnachtsmann* proclaim, *'Frohes Fest'*. In corners there are hanging stars, angels with trumpets, baskets of logs and twigs, thick fur rugs, sprigs of holly. *This* is the type of Christmas I want for Emily. I close my eyes and inhale deeply from the pine needles on the enormous tree, craving the scent's astonishing power to carry me back in time to childhood. When I open them I find it's my ten-year-old face reflected in a bauble. December will be magic again.

I put Emily in her high chair, then fetch her porridge from the kitchen. I've noticed she often holds her hands up, palms out; a gesture of surrender, then brings them down hard on the table. The sound invariably makes her laugh. She does this now, but she also takes the plastic spoon and places it in her mouth several times without it dropping. This is progress, and receives a round of applause. She's making an experimental consonant-vowel combination, too: *'Buh.'* A percussive utterance that maybe has as much to do with exploring sound as it does speech. I seize on any signs of development, imaginary or not.

After breakfast, I hold Emily up to the window again, and sing carols: 'O Come All Ye Faithful', 'God Rest Ye Merry Gentlemen', 'Silent Night'. She listens quietly, as if in church.

At midday, there is a traditional German Christmas dinner – goose, with *Kloß* (dumplings), creamy leek sauce, and *Rotkohl* (red cabbage). Emily is doted upon at the head of the table. I study her, sitting once again in her high chair. She gazes in awe at the bubbles rising in a glass of champagne. The endlessly replenishing tracer fire from the base of the flute to the lip fascinates her. She's as radiant as a queen, bathed in gold light from the candles.

Later, Anita and I take a walk with her, up the low hill visible from the lounge. It's a deserted, darkening winter's afternoon, Emily crying constantly in the buggy as we try to hold a conversation. When we reach the brow, Anita stops, mid-sentence. Emily's screaming stops, too. We breathe in the sharp air and listen to the murmuring of the leaves. Then we move on, the squeaking of the buggy's wheels the only other sound.

We've been talking continually about our daughter's development, the uncertainty hanging over us; the strain we're under. Anita took her to see a paediatrician here, before I arrived, and it wasn't a success, apparently. Although private and expensive, the meeting lasted a mere 15 minutes. The doctor was a sour man in his late fifties who made derisory remarks about the British healthcare system, and wouldn't be drawn on any treatment as it was 'against the rules', and he 'didn't know' our child. However, he did say we needed to find physiotherapy for Emily 'yesterday'. If a child in Germany had displayed Emily's symptoms, they would have received physiotherapy at three months, he assured.

So much crucial time has been lost, trying to secure appointments. We're still waiting to hear from Harefield House, even though the letter stated 'outcome accepted'. We may have to look for a private physio, I say.

The sun is sinking behind the mysterious forest, turning the trunks of the silver birch a lurid orange. A strange cast of light, like the supercharged moment just before a storm.

I turn to Anita and kiss her.

'I love you,' I say.

'I love you, too,' she replies. 'I haven't even had time to say that.'

We need to get away, I insist, stop being parents caught up in this bad dream; be ourselves. Book a weekend, anything. In all this, we've been neglecting each other.

The dark is thickening around us. You wouldn't want to be stranded out here at night. There are *Wildschwein* – wild boar – in the woods. They will attack, Anita's mother told me, especially if they feel their young are threatened. I know how they feel. We turn around, and begin to make our way back.

As we walk up the road to her parents' house, I put forward my theory about Dr McNally, why he seemed so cautious in the meeting. He's a medical man – and therefore a science man. He won't be hurried to any conclusions until all the results have been collated.

'I just wish there was one person who could reassure us,' Anita says. 'It feels like we're totally alone.'

7

Under Ice

BACK IN LONDON – on my own, to take advantage of work over New Year – I investigate Mumsnet. I've heard a lot about Mumsnet, but have never had the urge to consult it, until now. I type 'slow development' into the FAQs box, and a thread appears. Before long, there's ice in my stomach. One child was deprived of oxygen at birth, isn't walking at two years old, and has poor coarse and fine motor skills. 'Not walking after eighteen months is when to worry,' one parent writes. Well, Emily has less than four months to go. They all admit to suffering huge levels of stress and anxiety.

Some of the posts are deeply troubling. One mother is concerned because her daughter can only roll over from her back to tummy, can't crawl or walk, and 'playing' involves banging toys down and laughing at the sound. It could be a description of Emily. I note that the child is eight months old. Emily is 15 months. Then, for a moment, I feel ashamed. What if Emily had leukaemia, or a heart condition, instead of delayed development? What if we're worrying for nothing? We simply don't know.

The next day, a Siberian wind blows outside the flat, tugging at the bare branches of the copper beech. I make a Skype call to Anita in Germany. She tells me Emily had a private physiotherapy session yesterday, and it was an enormous success. I can hear an almost evangelical zeal in her voice: ' "The Bobath concept", a method that promotes motor learning, was employed. It's often used in cases of cerebral palsy.'

I fall silent.

'Don't panic,' says Anita.

Apparently, the therapist said that, with the correct treatment, Emily would soon be mobile. The happiness and relief in my wife's voice is infectious. I feel a surge of optimism: maybe we've found someone sympathetic to our daughter's needs.

New Year's Eve. It's dark outside, at 4pm. In the flat block opposite the house, Christmas tree lights, red and orange, glimmer behind curtains.

I'm missing Emily, and want to hold her in my arms as I pace around the lounge. I prepare plastic folders for her medical documents, and apply stickers to each: EEG, Physiotherapy, Bloods, Audiology, Genetics, MRI … I realise this is an attempt to render the frightening, rapidly evolving present safe. To classify it, archive it; pin it down somehow. I stack them up on the record player.

Should I play a record?

I think of the plan to listen only to new music. It seems trivial and pointless now; too much has changed since the autumn. I can't face listening to *any* music when my daughter's future is hanging in the balance. My beautiful, golden daughter. And anyway, it's time to leave for my gig.

The first week of January, a new year. Anita and I talk on Skype again about moving to Germany. We go over the advantages – and disadvantages – one more time. We have no day-to-day help with Emily, besides the nursery, and my brother, who visits one afternoon each week. Our respective parents live hundreds of miles away, my mother in Yorkshire, my father in Kent; Anita's in another country. We have no private pension, no life insurance, no savings. We are the last mugs in town, throwing money away on an inflated London rent, not even thinking about the future. (What about a second child?) Further, both of us feel trapped in our jobs. More and more teachers are leaving the profession, and it's easy to understand why. The risible salary, the endless target-driven assessments, the unpaid overtime. German teachers, according to Anita, earn twice as much, have civil servant status, drive BMWs, finish work at 1pm … A grass-is-greener dream perhaps, but still potent, nonetheless. Over there we could live cheaply, receive help from Anita's parents, maybe even save some money. Most importantly, Emily would receive prompt treatment from a well-funded health service. And I could write without having to do battle with London every week, something I'm now utterly weary of. Every penny of my income goes on rent, bills or the baby. It's almost Buddhist how I've snuffed out my desire for new possessions.

Privately, though, I'm fearful of how risky such a move could be. I agree in principle, but only for a couple of years. The UK is still my home. And not immediately, either: I need time to learn German, and find out if I can work over there.

In the weeks that follow, Emily's test appointments start to arrive. The EEG is first, in an unpleasantly hot room at St Mary's Children's Hospital. The nurse makes marks on our daughter's scalp with a special pencil, then applies glue, onto which electrodes are attached. Over these go a kind of hair net. Predictably, Emily loathes the procedure. She screams and howls, snot, tears and spit running down her enraged face.

But the following morning, with no hospital appointment to attend, Emily is happy as we rattle down Victoria Road on the freezing nursery run. Strapped into the buggy, wearing her plum-coloured cardigan and cream coat, and the purple mittens into which I can never fit her thumbs, she makes appreciative, cooing noises as we pass familiar faces.

A woman pushing a pram overtakes us. The little boy inside, about the same age as Emily, sees a 4x4 on the road, and his hand shoots out, index finger pointing.

'Ka!' he says. Car.

It strikes me that Emily has never pointed at a car. In fact, she's never pointed at anything, or followed my finger when I point. Why?

Two days later, I overhear Anita on the phone, speaking to a private physiotherapist we may be hiring. Her name is Jane, and she charges an eye-watering £95 an hour. They seem to have already bonded; my wife sounds as if she's talking with an old girlfriend.

'I can see Emily wants to move,' Anita says, '*needs* to move, but she can't. She's getting so frustrated.'

I hear the phrase 'Bobath concept'. Then timings being discussed, an appointment being booked.

A copy of the paediatrician's report arrives. It's many hours before I can face opening it. When I do, I read as quickly as I can, gulping down the information as if that way it will hurt less.

There's a list of the investigations proposed by Dr McNally in the meeting, followed by his clinical observations, and information supplied by us.

Emily has no problem with chewing or swallowing ...
Occasionally she has 'head drop' and stiffness in her body
... There is no skin abnormality and no symptoms or signs
to suggest neurocutaneous problems ... She is not crawling.
She has managed to weight bear but is not able to lift herself
up. Also, she is not exploring any toys, or sharing them ...
Parents say that she has got quite good eye contact with
them at home, and that she laughs and giggles ... Speech:
significant delay, with just babbling, no obvious words ...
Health-wise, Emily looks well in herself. There is no obvious
illness ... Emily is the first child for both parents. There
is no consanguinity ... She did not have good eye contact
with me at all in the clinic [underlined, for some reason]
... Sometimes Emily becomes stressed, cries and screams
... She did not have any ritual movement while in the
clinic ... Her chest, heart and abdominal examination are

*normal. Normal tone and reflexes of her upper and lower
limbs. Muscle mass is small on her lower limbs. Normal
cranial nerves. Normal oral examination, apart from a
high arched palette. No dysmorphic features ... Impression:
Global Developmental Delay, mainly social communication
disorder and gross motor delay. Urgent action: agreed
in discussion with the parents. She needs multiple
investigations. Review in three to six months time.*

I push the letter back into the envelope. It's shocking to see it
all in black and white. Although, in a way, the last sentence
about the follow-up appointment is reassuring. We've finally
connected to what we so ardently wished for: a medical
support network.

Yet, at the same time, I understand we're in very deep trouble.

*

'I think Emily might have Low Sensory Threshold. Babies with
LST don't move that much, don't help as much with their own
birth, hence the difficult labour.'

The speaker is Jane, the private physiotherapist, a compact,
friendly Australian woman in her late twenties. Anita and I
exchange a glance. This is a revelation. We're in the lounge, a
wet Thursday afternoon in January.

She continues: 'Low Sensory Threshold means they become
agitated at too much input. Some babies are just *yeah, yeah,
yeah*,' and she does a sort of contented, bobbing-along
impression that could be Billy, or any of the children at the
nursery, 'but some react more to sounds and visual stimuli.'

A memory leaps back. About six months ago, preparing food in the kitchen while Emily was in the lounge, I opened a cupboard, accidentally causing a deluge of steel pots and pans to fall crashing to the tiled floor, a tumultuous sound. Then I heard Emily burst into tears, real howls, as if she was in physical pain.

It all makes sense now. Yet I'm cautious, because I know I'm desperate for answers, easily led, and half mad with worry, but it really does. Why has no GP or paediatrician told us any of this?

We've been in the room for almost an hour. I'm sitting at the dining table, Anita on the playmat, Jane on the sofa. Emily is still in her bedroom, napping. We've related the whole story, from birth to present day, Jane listening intently.

'When you told me about the colic reflux, a light bulb went off,' she goes on. 'The Eustachian tubes in the ears are horizontal, so stomach acid, and milk, even, can get into their ears, causing congestion. That's why they say never feed a baby flat. If it doesn't drain properly it can be misdiagnosed as an ear infection. Children with severe reflux are in survival mode, and slower to be concerned with physical milestones. Basically, it meant she didn't have the "calm awake" state she needed to learn new skills.'

We're opened-mouthed. This woman is a marvel.

I tell Jane that the paediatrician has recommended an MRI brain scan. She grimaces slightly.

'I'd say, don't do it. Not at the moment, not with all her symptoms. It requires a general anaesthetic, and you don't want her to be the one-in-whatever-it-is that has an adverse reaction. And anyway, often an MRI can show scary things that don't manifest later. Their brains are still developing, they're plastic. It can show "damage" that isn't there.'

We can hear Emily waking up in the room next door. Anita rises, leaves the lounge, and a minute later brings our daughter in.

'Hello, missy!' says Jane. 'Gosh, how pretty are *you?*'

Emily, still in her pyjamas, her movements slow from sleep, is placed on the playmat. She seems quietly bemused, yet intrigued by this new person. A tentative smile appears on her face.

'What about her not responding to us pointing at things?' I ask. My questions seem to come from an endless source.

'Her receptive communication? That may come soon, hopefully,' Jane replies.

'And her "hands-up" stance?'

'It's called "high guard", or "fixing", to give her a sense of stability. They're faking core strength. And they can't point when they do that. It also goes back to the reflux, stuck in a pain stance.'

'The bashing on the table?'

'She might think, I'll bash so I create sensory impressions.'

Jane crouches down next to Emily to study her movements. 'Hmm,' she says, 'she certainly follows the path of least resistance.' I notice she is tender, yet assured with her. 'You're going to have to work hard with me, missy!'

The session is concluding. Jane suggests that Emily doesn't have hypotonia, but maybe she is hypermobile – double-jointed, in layman's terms.

She examines Emily's face. 'Hmm, in true Global Developmental Delay, teeth are late, and the ears are low. I'm not *that* worried about her …'

'One last question,' I say, 'why is it called "Global" Developmental Delay?'

'It just means that the delays are across the board; that all her skills – learning to walk or talk, or interacting with others socially and emotionally – will take longer.'

We walk Jane to the stairs; I hand over £95 in cash. As she gathers her coat and boots, she smiles, 'But we need to get her upper body to twist first. Core turns. That's what we'll start on in the next session!'

When she's gone, Anita turns to me, exalted.

'You know that one person we talked about on the walk at my parents', the one person who could reassure us,' she says. 'It's her.'

I watch Jane from the high window in the lounge, striding across the rain-lashed street to her parked car. I would have paid twice her fee.

The next day, at the nursery, I tell Laura – the young Scottish manager – that Emily has Global Developmental Delay. The words sound grand and terrifying as they leave my mouth. A nervous expression appears on her face, similar to the one worn by my fellow band members that time at the gig in Covent Garden. But she recovers quickly, and says that she and her co-workers will do anything they can to help, 'in our small way'.

*

Hope. It's an exhausting word, hope. Hope is the thing with feathers, as Emily Dickinson wrote, that perches in the soul and sings the tune without words – and never stops, at all. I'm *hoping* that Emily's development is latent, that some command centre in her brain will start sending its messages soon, and she will be released into life. I'm hoping that, before long, she'll be able to walk, to run, to speak like the others. Yet I realise I've mentally shut down all those hopes I had for her future, just in case they never happen. Riding a bike, building a snowman, learning an instrument, buying make-up and travelling with friends, a career, a marriage ... A life. I didn't intend this to happen, it just has. It gives me a feeling of intense sadness. I live from day to day with no idea if there will be a 'happy ending'. By October, when she is two, will Emily have caught up with the others? I wonder constantly what they are up to, the NCT kids, and feel a deep, bitter envy at them, forging ahead.

I'm hoping for a time when these feelings stop.

The following weekend, walking by the river to Kingston with Emily in the buggy, Anita and I discuss who does the best animal noises for her. My cow's moo is better than her frog rivet, but her monkey, I have to concede, pisses all over my monkey. It's a nature-documentary perfect 'ooh ooh-*ah ah*', a binary call rising on the two *ahs*. It's very accomplished, I say.

'Well, that's three years of teaching five-year-olds for you,' Anita says. 'I had a school friend once who could do a great horse's neigh.'

'Really?'

'Yes, and she could fold her ear lobe into her ... I don't know what you'd call it. Ear hole?'

'Wow. Quite some skillset. I expect she's a high-flyer now.'

'She did a brilliant lawnmower, too. Perfect,' she says.

'Well if I ever need an equine impersonator contortionist, I'll look her up.'

'She couldn't burp the alphabet, though, like me.'

'That's because you had an older brother. You and I used to have serious conversations, you know.'

'No, that's the thing,' she says, stopping and turning to me. 'It's all too serious at the moment.'

'I know. I hope Em does something soon,' I say.

'I think she will. I *know* she will.'

I've been singing the Beatles' 'Mother Nature's Son' to Emily at bedtime. It seems to calm her; the long, even metre of the opening notes sound madrigal-like when sung a cappella. I do this while brushing her teeth: me sitting on the edge of the bath, her tiny body perched upon my knees. She opens her mouth like a cuckoo, makes a soft sound of appreciation – *ah* – as she tastes the minty toothpaste. Sometimes she copies a note, and I pat my hand over her mouth to make a sort of holler: *wo wo wo wo wo*. It makes her laugh, but then I realise it's the only reciprocal thing she does, and I feel panic.

After I've put her to bed, I contemplate playing an album. The plan to listen to new music – while keeping a record of Emily's milestones – has been a dismal failure, and I decide to quietly abandon it.

At the weekend, I read in the paper that novelist Henning Mankell couldn't read new books after his cancer diagnosis, only the ones he'd loved all his life. And so I decide, from now on, to listen only to the old music.

8

The Colour
of Spring

WHEN I WAS 17, my favourite band was Talk Talk. Once a moderately successful early-eighties British synth-pop outfit, they had evolved, during a short space of time, into something rather different. The LP they released that year, 1986, *The Colour of Spring*, was experimental, melancholy, and, in stark contrast to their earlier incarnation – and most of the rest of the charts – featured many 'real' instruments.

With late January becoming almost spring-like, I look for my vinyl copy of the record. It seems to have vanished, so I search YouTube, and find Tim Pope's video for my favourite tune on the album, the big single, 'Life's What You Make It'. I click 'play'. A tight close-up of a piano keyboard appears, just the black notes – huge, polished leviathans reflecting a ghostly, blueish light. Silence. A bug – a woodlouse, perhaps – clambers over the edge of one, a tiny mountaineer. There is still no sound, just a background thrum of what could be insects in a forest at night.

Boom!

The track bursts into life. A wide shot reveals a shadowy figure in dark glasses and a suede jacket with turned-up collars: the pianist. He's struck the first note of the riff at precisely the same moment as the first kick-drum hit. Shivers of pleasure tingle across my upper back and neck. A starburst guitar figure, impossibly high in the mix, explodes from out of nowhere. A scorching, 1960s Hammond organ emerges in the backing layers. The music – with its peculiar blend of optimism and regret – speaks to me as it did when I first heard it in the bedroom of my father's house, after my parents' separation. I'm a teenager again: full of restless, youthful enthusiasm, but with a strange core of anxiety.

We see the drummer next: intense, pony-tailed, playing along to a programmed pattern, yet hitting the skins immensely hard, putting his entire bodyweight into the action. And yes, they are indeed outdoors, at night, in a forest. There are moon shadows. It's cold: there's condensation on his drums.

Cutaway shots reveal wildlife: a glossy centipede crawls – filling the screen; a white owl takes flight, a fox startles. We see these creatures as a child might see them, close-up, for the first time. The colours seem to reference the English 19th-century painter Samuel Palmer, who painted rural night-time scenes: rich blues, muted greens, gleaming silvers.

The pianist is also the singer, and his breath comes out in a cloud as he sings the first word:

Baby …

And I suddenly recall how thrilling this pop locution was in such a serious piece of work. He follows it with the title of the song: 'Life's What You Make It'. But what I really loved at 17 was the simplicity of every element, the unerring repetition, the same riff and lyric over and over. The piano motif and vocal melody consist of only a handful of notes, endlessly recycled. The drummer plays no fills at all, a pattern reminiscent of Kate Bush's 'Running Up That Hill', but also – since I'm now familiar with the 1970s German bands – Can's *Tago Mago*.

Towards the halfway mark, massed backing vocals reassure that everything will be 'all right'. It is the only time a band member – bassist Paul Webb – looks directly into the camera. As the song fades, a pale, misty dawn is coming up, rabbits hop among the ferns.

Suitably ravished, I decide to look for my other favourite on *The Colour of Spring*, the quiet song that ends side one, a tune that I came back to again and again as a shy, introspective teenager. 'April 5th' seems at odds with the rest of the record, yet somehow integrated. A beginning rather than an ending. It is a fragile, impressionistic piece, the song in which Talk Talk accidentally stumble upon their luminous new sound, explored later on the final two albums, *Spirit of Eden* and *Laughing Stock*. A realisation must have occurred that a tiny brushstroke, a shiver of guitar, or feedback, could produce a huge effect.

I find the clip, and press 'play'. A dobro acoustic chimes, a swish of percussion repeats. The music proceeds haltingly, suggesting the incremental onset of spring. The vocal – in which it is hard to make out many words – expresses frustration, impatience. The first unformed utterances of a child. And this is why I'm playing it now, and will play it obsessively in the days to come, watching Emily on her playmat, trying to find the path ahead.

February. A new month. Emily's physiotherapy exercises nearly always cause her to cry. They must hurt, or at least she might feel the burn, as in a workout. They're distressing to watch. I sit her on the floor, holding her lower down, around the pelvis, as any higher up lends too much assistance. Then, with a toy as an incentive, I gently push her forward into a fall – a core turn to produce a saving reaction with both hands. This will result in a weight-bearing position, and is first base for a child to start crawling. They need to be on 'four points', in physiotherapy jargon – all fours. Invariably, though, she extends her legs until she is almost standing. This isn't much use, as they are stiff and straight. It's the bend at the knee that is the springboard.

I explain that we must get her core strong or she'll never be able to crawl or walk. She lies on her front, flapping her hands, back arched like a bow. 'Are you trying to fly, tiny Bear?' I ask. It will start to look odd soon, I think to myself, this toddler just lying there in the nursery, not crawling.

We will try again later. I pick up the acoustic guitar and start playing songs for her. Blues and rock'n'roll. Fats Domino's 'I'm Walkin'', Chuck Berry's 'You Never Can Tell', Johnny Cash's 'Folsom Prison Blues', Elvis's 'That's Alright (Mama)'. She suddenly becomes thoughtful, attentive. For the first time, I notice she's curious about the instrument itself. I let her touch the strings, around the sound-hole. She starts yanking at them clumsily with her fingers. Then she bashes the top of the guitar with open palms, transfixed by the hollow sound, and how it changes in pitch depending on where her hands impact. She switches the action to the strings. Discreetly, I fret a chord with my left hand. An open C, then an F barre. I start singing the Rolling Stones's 'You Can't Always Get What You Want'. (An apt choice, perhaps.) I time the changes to her strikes, and slowly, surely, the progression starts to emerge. I to IV, I to IV. The blues. She's 'playing' the guitar. I check her reaction. She's smiling.

But the truth is, I'm feeling the strain at the moment. She cries so much more than the other NCT children. They make their parents' lives easier by being able to play with a toy for long periods of time. Emily simply cannot do this. Sometimes it overwhelms me, watching her sitting on the floor with the heavy plinth that holds the plastic hoops, screaming, bashing it down then throwing it aside, over and over again. Suddenly, I feel anger and disappointment towards my daughter, as if she's let me down somehow. *Why can't you just bloody play with it properly, like Billy does?* I find myself thinking. And then, of course, I'm engulfed with shame for having such a thought.

*

'When do you think she will walk?' asks Anita. We're in the kitchen, late one February afternoon, preparing pizza and salad.

'Two, if that.' I reply, staring out of the window at the red glare of a sunset. It looks as if there's a fire inside one of the opposite flats. I can't seem to conceal my pessimism anymore.

'I think it'll be earlier than that,' she says.

Anita seems cheerful again, has been humming tunes around

the flat over the past few days. This lifts my spirits, although I can't be sure what's really in her mind.

We've been going over and over the questions again. Does Emily understand when you ask her something? Clearly no, and at her age, this is deeply worrying. I recall Andrew with Billy on holiday: *Where's your nose, Billy?* A pause, then he pointed to it. He couldn't *say* the word nose, but he knew what one was.

'It's her basic comprehension that's missing,' I say, 'her … cognition.'

There's a parents' evening coming up at the nursery, says Anita.

'What will we talk about?'

'The curriculum.'

'The *curriculum?* Em is one.'

'Yes, there are five areas of development.'

'It'll be a short meeting then.'

She sends me a look.

I try to explain that I'm hanging on in hope, waiting for the green shoots of our daughter's development to appear. Waiting for the colour of spring.

But *are* some green shoots beginning to show? Emily's 'word' – *Beh!* – is becoming more pronounced. I imagine she is trying to say 'Bear'.

'Bear?' I ask. 'Where bear? There Bear!' pointing at her.

And when Anita returns from work one afternoon, she has a variation: *Bah!*

After a few attempts, she links two together.

Bah-Bah!

We exchange incredulous looks. Does this count as her first word? What could it be? Ba-Ba? Pa-Pa?

Papa.

We're back in the kitchen one evening when an extraordinary event occurs. Anita is holding Emily when, with no expectations, I say: 'Clap hands, Emily.'

And she does.

Her tiny, chubby hands connect. Once, twice. We stare at each other for a split-second, then explode, like football fans after a goal.

Emily seems confused; stops clapping. But this is huge, monumental. This is a milestone. This is hope. She can finally perform an action that her contemporaries were able to do last summer. Not only is it an example of motor skills in use, and evidence that her balance is improving – the high guard stance has to be relaxed to clap – it's a comprehension of a vocal prompt. I feel as if I've made contact at last with some distant life form. And this is the thing, this is what has been troubling me, a thought I haven't been able to share with anyone. If she can't understand language, then she is … not human, somehow. Yes, she has a spirit and a soul, of course she does, but language makes us human, surely. She recognises us visually, but pets recognise their owners. Now, in my mind, she's crossed the line from animal to human.

'You understand!' I yell, punching the air, leaping up and down. Emily looks embarrassed. But I'm elated.

She's going to be all right.

Dr McNally calls me one morning, unexpectedly. I've been chasing him, leaving messages with his secretary. The EEG and the bloods are both normal. Thyroid, enzymes, creatine – all normal.

'So if the bloods and the other tests are fine,' I say, 'the problems are …?'

'Related to the brain.'

I feel a stab of the old terror. My arms feel suddenly cold.

He continues: 'These things can correct themselves, but we can't move to the next step without the MRI.'

He's still pushing. I allow an uneasy silence to grow.

'I know you and your wife are still discussing it,' he goes on, 'but if Emily is not improving, the MRI needs to be done.'

'What about the genetic tests?' I ask.

'Well, yes, but they take a long time and are very involved. I won't explain here, because you'll become confused.'

Try me, I think.

He continues, 'When they see Emily they will suggest which tests need to be done.'

Then I hear a smile enter his voice. 'Carry on as normal, you and your wife. Try not to worry about your daughter. Enjoy her. It's one step at a time at the moment.'

I put down the phone and attempt to breathe. I check my email. He's sent the blood test results as requested, a bewildering full-colour NHS spreadsheet.

Later, walking back with Emily from the nursery, I stare at her small plump hands emerging from the buggy, the marbling of the veins just below the skin. I think of the complexity of the human system; what is carried in her blood and what can be inferred from it. And at the centre, pumping it around her body, her little heart, the engine that carries her through each night, asleep in her room.

'The normal blood enzyme is a good thing. It confirms she doesn't have hypotonia, which can result from a brain injury, and is degenerative.'

Jane again, the second physiotherapy session in the lounge. Anita and I are discussing the test results with her. She advises us not to be impatient with the genetic investigations; they can go on for years. Blood has to be taken first, then, if necessary, a surgical biopsy: an incision into the thigh. Anita winces. I imagine the knife, Emily's poor leg ...

Jane has some new exercises for her. A sort of cushion ramp leading up to the sofa, to stimulate crawling. She informs us that Emily is overusing her extensors – 'arching with that double-jointed spine of hers' – and this intervention will help. We run through several assisted laps. I hold onto Emily's tiny waist as she grips the cushion on four points, looking from side to side, her big grey-blue eyes absorbed in the curious novelty of the act. Then, when she's steady, I push her knees forward, one at a time. As she reaches the summit, she collapses from the effort and I help her slip clumsily to the floor. We repeat the exercise. Then we do it again. And again.

As the session concludes, Jane announces she's pleased with the slight progress on show.

'I don't go home at night and worry about Emily,' she says. 'Yes, she's delayed, but ...'

She notices our searching, anxious expressions, and becomes

uncomfortable. The three of us are standing in the middle of the room, Anita and I with our arms crossed, eager to hear any words of comfort. We must look like children waiting for a parent to reassure us that everything will be all right, that the big bad wolf has gone away.

'But she's improving. Slowly.'

*

A cold February morning. Yet by lunchtime it is almost spring-like. Crocuses are pushing through in Claremont Gardens; some blossom already out. We have another appointment at the hospital, Emily's hip X-ray. More tests. And more to come, I think wearily.

We still don't have all the pieces of the puzzle.

*

Normal. I have been brooding on the word normal, and its antonym, abnormal. Jane became flustered the other day when she referred to a 'normal' child in comparison to Emily. She quickly corrected herself: 'I hate to use the word normal, but …' And just last week, when we rushed Emily to A&E with a high fever, the young, female doctor discussing the tests began, 'Because your child isn't developing normally …' and I saw a shadow of misgiving pass over her eyes as she spoke, but it was soon gone. She was a busy emergency doctor, after all, with more pressing concerns than hurting a parent's feelings. But even so, it feels as if Emily is slowly beginning to be moved to the other side of normal.

Abnormal.

This is what you see when you enter Church Passage from Claremont Road: a wide path on a gentle incline that seems to stop abruptly after about ten metres. Here, by a streetlight, the alley bends sharply to the left, and branches from adjacent gardens form an arbour. It's at this spot I pause on my midnight walk home from work, and take a rest. I put the guitar bag down; exhale. Our building becomes visible here, and I have a warm feeling, knowing that Emily is safe, asleep in her bedroom at the top of the house.

There is whispering in my ears. Cocteau Twins' 'Otterly', from their album *Treasure*, is on the iPod. (I'm listening to the old music again, teenage favourites: everything from the Beatles to Nick Drake. And, especially, at the moment, the Cocteaus.) Singer Elizabeth Fraser's vocal consists entirely of incomprehensible whispers, over an amniotic wash of sea effects. Sometimes you can make out a word, but it's clear you aren't meant to, merely respond to its sound on an emotional level.

I breathe in deeply for a moment, assimilate my surroundings. An unmanageable ivy bush growing on top of a garden shed spills over the path. A section of wall bows and bulges, pushed out by tree roots. Vertical strips of metal have been screwed in place to prevent it from crumbling.

If I was to walk on, the spire of St Mark's would appear, but I remain motionless, absorbing the scene. Steam issues from my mouth; it's cold, it's late, but I'm unable to move. Early tomorrow morning, I will charge down here with the buggy, in bright spring sunlight, the gardens beyond the walls ablaze with colour, blackbirds watching us with orange-rimmed eyes.

But tonight it vibrates with a different energy. It is a charged, uncanny place. Nimble foxes run the fences, and cats patrol the gardens. I wonder if Emily dreams of buckling brickwork, and ivy on old walls. Of blackbirds and cats and quick, cunning foxes. I don't know – she hasn't been able to tell me yet. She sees the world, I watch her respond to it with such sensitivity, and – I believe – intelligence, but she can't or won't comment.

The ivy is shifting now with almost imperceptible movements, and I try to grasp its pattern; its mystery, what English 20th-century landscape painter Paul Nash called 'things behind'.

I feel a droplet hit my face. Looking up, I see it's starting to rain. A blur of fast drizzle shows, illuminated below the streetlight, like static on an old television picture. I heave the guitar bag over my shoulder, and walk the last steps home.

Emily is 16 months old. Out of sheer frustration, I decide that she *will* crawl. I set her on the playmat, put her in the first base position, and move her forward: one knee and one hand at a time. But she soon collapses – there's too little strength in her legs, her sagging back – and she ends up face down, arms flailing.

I try some side-sitting exercises with her instead. These are even less encouraging. Her struggle to move into the crawling position from a seated start; the helpless movements of her knees, like those of a newborn foal, are pitiful to watch. She starts crying – tears of frustration – and reaches for my hand to pull her up to a stand. I stroke her back. Don't worry, my darling, we'll try again tomorrow.

We drive to Harefield House for a meeting with the community paediatrician. It's a fine afternoon, the church spire on Ewell Road gilded with sunshine, the daffodils out a month early. Daffodils are *Osterglocken* in German – Easter bells. How much more poetic than the rather limp English word.

As we pull into the car park, Anita warns me: 'You may see some things that will upset you.' This is, after all, the 'Centre for children with disabilities', the words from the letterhead that punched me in the stomach back in December. I carry Emily into the building over my shoulder, steeling myself for terrible sights. We share a lift with a boy in tartan pyjamas, slumped, dribbling, in a large pushchair. He must be about 15 or 16. In the waiting room, a kid no older than ten sits with his dad. He wears a red pullover, is gap-toothed and has something odd about his eyes. The boy can't seem to keep his hands still, they twist and flap in his lap.

Jane appears, all Antipodean optimism and efficiency, and we are led to the consulting room. There are five female medical professionals waiting to receive us: the senior paediatrician, seated behind her desk; another, younger doctor; a speech therapist; a second physiotherapist, and Jane. I experience a dizzy sensation close to vertigo. All these people are here for us, for Emily's problems. It somehow deepens the seriousness of the situation.

The room is oppressively hot, and soon everyone has red cheeks. There is a palpable atmosphere of sympathy, however; we're surrounded by kind, concerned expressions. Emily is relaxed, and pleasantly stimulated by the new faces. She's set down on a playmat, on which a giant space battle is taking place.

The paediatrician begins with the expected volley of questions:

'Does she pretend to use a spoon?'

'No.'

'A toy phone?'

'No.'

Etc., etc.

Then she crosses the room, crouches down before Emily, and tries to interest her in some small, colourful cubes. She waves a wand containing fairy dust, holds it high to see if Emily follows it with her eyes. After several more tests using various toys there is a physical examination. She pulls down Emily's tights to assess her muscle tone. Then her reflexes are tested with a miniature wooden hammer.

During this, I hold an intermittent conversation with Jane, who is sitting beside me, watching closely. I tell her that Emily clapped her hands on request, but won't do it anymore. Should we be worried? This is normal, she says. All skills are in competition. She will put aside an old one as a new one is learned. We discuss Emily's low sensory threshold again. She reminds me that her sensory starting point was always over-stimulated because of the colic reflux. I tax her with more questions; they seem to tumble out in a never-ending stream. It is here that I realise Jane truly has become our confidante, our confessor.

The speech therapist takes over, attempts to talk to Emily. I interrupt her with queries and ideas from my notebook, things that have been troubling me for months. I find I'm trying to control the meeting, talking too much, yet powerless to stop myself. After a while, I notice all enquiries are being addressed to 'Mum'.

The therapist suggests we cut out the 'filler' words. Just say 'coat?' instead of 'Shall we find your coat?' Or 'banana?' rather than 'Would you like a banana?' Use repetitions, simple nouns.

The paediatrician, back at her desk, has completed the assessment. She shows us a form with many ticked boxes, and begins to explain what each one means. After a lengthy summing-up, she informs us that Emily has the developmental age of an eight- to ten-month-old.

I feel as if I've been punched in the stomach again.

But she's on her way to being two, not *eight- to ten months*. That's – what – last June?

She continues: Emily will need an occupational therapist, a speech therapist, and 'Portage' to teach her how to play.

Our time is up. A follow-up meeting is scheduled for six months. I gather our coats, bags, hats, toys, half-eaten snacks and used wet wipes, and we're shown out courteously.

Back home, in the kitchen, Anita seems oddly buoyant. 'I think our *Kleine Supermaus* will be just fine,' she says, warming the milk in the microwave.

I smile weakly, but I can see dark clouds gathering.

9

Pearly-Dewdrops' Drops

THREE DAYS OF rare March sunshine. I see forward motion everywhere. The flat is overrun with ladybirds – they move fast, upside down on window frames, or slowly across the polished wooden floors. Outside, children leap about in Long Ditton rec, walk together in school outing lines. Brown-eyed girls zip past on micro-scooters. And on the Tube, an advertisement tagline for Wellbaby catches my eye:

For the start of their journey!

Forward motion everywhere, except on the playmat.

The invasive tests keep coming. The eye examination is the worst. The nurse holds a screaming Emily in a headlock, administering drops to dilate her pupils. We look on in horror. But it turns out her vision is excellent. The audiology investigation, however, does reveal something: she has a build-up of fluid, or 'glue ear', probably as a result of her many infections. At the moment, she is partially deaf, 'as if she's walking around with her fingers in her ears,' in the doctor's words. And this confuses matters: is her speech delay because of reduced hearing, or merely aggravated by it? Could the glue ear explain why she never responds to her name?

The final pieces of the puzzle are being assembled, yet somehow not fitting together. There is only one more test left before the MRI: genetics.

One morning I find Anita stirring porridge in the kitchen, tears in her eyes. She tells me the nursery has suggested they find Emily a council-funded one-to-one helper. This is the first step towards a Special Educational Needs classification, she says, and our daughter will become labelled as 'Special'. But she does have actual 'special needs', I venture. (For once, it's me trying to reassure her; we seem to have changed places.) As the nursery staff gently pointed out, Emily spends most of her time there in the Float Baby Bouncer, crying. Her contemporaries can all crawl or walk, and will soon move upstairs to the over-twos room. Emily will be left with a new intake of babies. And she's not a baby anymore.

There is something troubling me, however. I know the nursery will receive more money from the council with a one-to-one in their employ, and maybe this is their motive. In my current fretful state, I've become mistrustful, paranoid. I see agendas and subterfuge everywhere; people against us. Conspiracy theories.

I need to get out. I grab my coat and keys, and make my way briskly through the cold, grey streets of the town to a cafe where I sometimes write. When I push through the doors, Italian pop is on the radio. I have a flashback to Sardinia. Simpler times.

At the first table is a dad, sitting with his young son, taking pleasure in the boy's easy play with a toy aeroplane. He notices me staring, and gives me a sharp look. I turn away, ashamed of how envious I am of them both.

Walking up Church Passage one April morning, shopping bag in hand, I notice a bright spray of daffodils has appeared in our high kitchen window. A symbolism all too neat, perhaps, for today there are signs of progress. Emily's assisted walking is becoming faster, surer. What's more, she can now play a 'game'. She waits as I place brightly coloured balls, or the plastic hoops on a low table, then she pushes them off with both hands. The sound as they hit the floor delights her, makes her giggle. I pick up the objects, put them back on the surface, and we repeat the game. I realise, with sadness, it's the first time she's actually played with anything. Yet I am hopeful about this interaction with me – she seems to keenly anticipate the toys being replaced before the next turn. It's a shared activity. There is communication, of a sort, between us.

Later, when she's settled for her nap, I attempt to do some admin. Emily's hospital paperwork is out of control. There is so much of it, sitting on top of the record player, defying all attempts at organisation. Old appointments, cancelled appointments; a letter informing us we didn't attend an unnecessary audiology appointment at St Mary's. I phoned four times on the morning to say we couldn't come, out of respect for the NHS, then waited on hold for 15 minutes, before giving up. A confused voice periodically broke through: *Switchboard?* Sometimes I fear the system is actually close to collapse.

It's two days later. I stand motionless in the doorway of the lounge as if witnessing a miracle. I *am* witnessing a miracle. Emily, unaware of me, is attempting to raise herself from the side-sitting position to all fours. Slowly, tremblingly, using all her strength, she tries to shift her weight.

Ah! she cries.

She's done it. She's on four points, ready to crawl. I'm not breathing. All I can hear is the faint sound of traffic on Claremont Road. When she finally collapses onto her front, I burst in, cheering wildly. *You did it!* Then I crawl rapidly around the room, to demonstrate how it should be done, which, of course, she finds hysterical. I put her back into the first position, and start to text Anita, when she repeats the manoeuvre. I go berserk, leaping up and down, praising her. I'm in heaven – she's learning to crawl.

Finally. Finally.

I begin to film her on my phone as she repeats the sequence of movements. She starts confidently, but then falls backwards. I'm too slow to catch her, and her head connects with the floor. Luckily, there was a soft-toy hedgehog on the wooden boards. Enough, I tell myself. Don't ask for more. This is a breakthrough.

The next evening, Anita is at an after-school event, and I'm solo with Emily. I feed her yoghurt with strawberries, followed by full-fat Philadelphia cheese on dense Swiss bread. Then, after the bath, I search for a book, but decide against it. I no longer read to her, I realise. I stopped when it became like an early Beatles concert, the screaming drowning out the words.

Instead, I play songs for her on the guitar. She's in good spirits, there are hardly any tears. Finally, when she's drunk her milk, I walk over to the stereo and take an album from the shelf: Talk Talk's *The Colour of Spring*. I finally located it. She loves playing peek-a-boo with vinyl records. I cover my face with the disc, look through the hole and see her grinning. I lower the needle onto side one's last track, 'April 5th'. Her face – so perfect in every way – turns to watch. I notice how the light strikes the planes of it, how she is endlessly, magnetically watchable, like the great film stars.

The tune drifts from the speakers, fragments of sound. What is Hollis singing? One word, repeated over and over. It sounds like *breakthrough*. I always thought it was *let me*, but now I'm certain it is *breakthrough*.

Breakthrough.

The emotions it stirs are oceanic. Helpless tears run down my face. Emily, an uncertain smile on her lips, considers her father with mild curiosity. I'm glad she won't remember this.

'Daddy's not sad,' I manage to say, stupidly. 'He's happy – happy, happy, happy.'

*

I'm called to a midday meeting at the nursery. Laura, and a woman from the council, would like to talk about Emily's one-to-one helper. I don't take off my coat – I'm in a suspicious, defensive mood after discussing the matter with Anita, and intending to make it a brief conversation. Plus, I have to pick up Emily from the downstairs crèche in 15 minutes.

The council lady wears a boxy, shoulder-padded jacket,

and a small, antique watch on her left wrist. Disconcertingly, she emits a high, flute-y laugh after she says anything contentious, or likely to startle a parent. Such as: 'Of course, we don't know what the future holds!' – i.e. Emily may not develop normally at all. She uses this phrase three times during the meeting, followed by the strange, inappropriate, nervous-tic giggle.

Laura sits opposite me, a concerned look on her face. I speak too much, eager to demonstrate my recently acquired, half-digested physiotherapy knowledge: 'high guard', 'calm, awake state', 'extensors'. All the while, I'm aware of the woman's notes in a folder before us on a low table. *Emily 1, Emily 2.* They cause desperate feelings in me. That it has come to this.

She explains that, in addition to one-to-one help, they offer everything from emotional support counsellors to specially built chairs to DLA. (I have to ask what this means – it stands for Disability Living Allowance.) *Of course, we don't know what the future holds!* We settle on two hours for Emily each nursery morning, overseen at first by Jane. I'm hot in my coat by now, and anxious to collect my daughter. I draw the meeting to a close, and make my way downstairs, reflecting briefly on the conversation. Maybe I could have been less curt with them. I still see hidden agendas everywhere. Perhaps the nursery really *are* behind us.

I find the crèche in its usual state of post-morning chaos. Ripe smells of food and faeces assail me. I struggle to put a squirming Emily into her cream coat, while listening with one ear to the key worker's summary – what she ate, how long she napped, trying to absorb some of it. When we're ready, she waves goodbye to Emily, quacking like a duck for her to elicit a reaction. Emily grins. Yes, they would all do anything to see one of her smiles.

Pushing the buggy past the line of pollarded plane trees on Balaclava Road, moments from the meeting return. Laura expressed concern about Emily's eye contact. 'She doesn't respond to me,' she said, with a serious, almost pained expression. I replied: 'That's probably because she's half deaf from glue ear, and when you do get eye contact, it's pretty good.' She nodded furiously. But then I remember Jane was concerned about Emily's 'absences', too. Moments when she waved her hand in front of her eyes. *Hello?* Nothing. She seemed to be zoning out. Maybe she's having seizures? But her EEG was fine. It still worries me, though. None of this will be resolved until we find out if everything is all right with her brain. And that means the MRI.

Today is the first official day of spring. I work with Emily on her exercises in the living room. Despite her recent breakthrough, progress is painfully slow. She raises herself to a sort of press-up, then curls a leg underneath her body in an attempt to find a kneeling position. But she soon collapses, onto her stomach, beating the floor with her tiny fists in rage. I set up the cushion ramp for her instead. She orientates herself towards it – an encouraging sign – but this takes all her strength; grizzling, clawing at the textured surface of the playmat with her nails in frustration.

I take her from the lounge to another room, to break state. A hiding and tickling session. She loves it when I crouch behind the bed, then leap, cartoon-frog style; adores being rolypolyed. She giggles, squeals, *screams* with delight. She is happy, extravagantly happy. And so am I. Time and place evaporate. I forget that I have a name, even. All is erased, suspended in the pure moment of play.

A curious thing happens on the way back from nursery. Emily is in her customary subdued state, as if the fun is over for another day, and there is nothing to look forward to anymore. I can never reach her when she is like this, so I push the buggy, while singing songs or talking to her. But this time I take a different route, via the shops – we desperately need nappies – and she starts to cry. Real, howling, anguished sobs. I have to stop and dry her face. Mothers, workmen with wheelbarrows, truants – all stare at us. I don't know what the matter is. I even consider leaving the buggy in some alley and carrying her home. She's not ill; I checked her temperature before we left. It's only when we're pushing up Church Passage, on the final stretch home, that her crying stops, and I realise the cause might have been the alternative route. We take exactly the same roads back each time. So she really *is* sensitive to her surroundings, then. At the front door, I pass our downstairs neighbour, Anna, the Italian mother of two. I tell her what has just happened. She nods and says, 'They're far cleverer than we think!' I agree, but I know there is something else going on with Emily.

Carrie visits with little Billy. I haven't seen them since the holiday. Billy is not so little anymore, and is 'just naughty all the time', according to his mum. I long to have a naughty child. A naughty child is one that can move about. I go upstairs to the mezzanine to write, and listen gloomily to the conversation. Billy has words now.

'Apple'. 'Spider'. 'Car!'

Carrie, who is half-German, has taught him the translations, too.

Apfel. Spinne. Auto!

Later, I watch them walk up Church Hill Road, Billy in his yellow Gap Kids coat, hi-top trainers, one hand pushing his micro-scooter, the other held by his mother. After a few moments, Carrie lets go of it. I feel a lurch in my stomach: he's going to fall. Then I remember, he's not Emily, he can walk perfectly well on his own.

Later still, as evening falls, I'm upstairs again in the mezzanine. Anita is holding Emily up to the lounge window, pointing to the street below. They don't know I'm watching them.

'*Auto*,' Anita says. 'Brrm, brrm.'

Emily doesn't respond.

'*Auto*,' she repeats.

My beautiful wife and child.

Easter Sunday. We drive to a Richmond pub in changeable weather: a hysterical rainstorm, then, when we emerge from the car, sunshine; the trees washed, dazzling and dripping in the noon light. Somewhere a church bell chimes 12.

We're here for lunch with friends of ours, a couple with a son a few months older than Emily. Once we've ordered, I tell the father, Martin – a teacher – that our daughter has Global Developmental Delay (I'm eager to have it out of the way as soon as possible). His pupils widen, and his face, in three-quarter profile, becomes very still. Steady eye contact is maintained. This, I'm beginning to find, is the control other mums and dads automatically use when the subject is broached: they think they are about to be told something dreadful about a child. Afterwards, they will hold their own just that little bit closer. I realise I'm becoming inured to our unique (it feels unique, are we the only ones?) situation. Everyone else is just getting on with being parents – a tough enough job – normal development a given.

We move on to the safer waters of Emily's glue ear. Martin admits to having had the condition as a child; he needed grommets – surgically implanted tubes in the eardrum to drain fluid. His parents and teachers didn't know what the problem was at first, he wasn't responding to language.

'They thought I was a Special!' he says, and my stomach knots.

His son is clambering happily around on the banquette seating behind us. I ask when his boy began crawling. 'I don't know,' he grins, 'eight months? He just started. Now he's like a little bulldozer!'

I like Martin, but I feel bruised by this exchange.

Emily is becoming tired, and I take her outside to walk around, singing 'Row Your Boat'. Saliva drips from her mouth, and hangs over her bottom lip until a swift tissue is administered. She hates it, jerks her head from left to right. Then I carry her to the front of the pub and we watch a hailstorm demolish the street. She is transfixed by the rocks as they smash down onto the tarmac, or bounce madly on car roofs, crackling like roasting chestnuts. Above our heads, through tiny, tinny speakers, Otis

Redding sings 'My Girl'. It is an almost too-perfect moment, holding my daughter in my arms.

We return to our table, which by now is strewn with unfinished plates of fish and chips, semi-demolished burgers, half-drunk pints, tissues, crayons, wet wipes and dummies. The pub has filled with families. A newborn feeds under a shawl. Damp prams steam in corners, or clutter the path to the kitchen. A familiar Sunday scene that is being played out all over the country. We talk about possibly leaving London for Germany. Everyone is bailing out, it seems: they have their eye on the East Sussex coast.

Finally, we gather our belongings and head for the cars. Sunshine prevails once more. We say our goodbyes, and drive away, Emily asleep in the back. She has a new, larger seat now. She's growing.

I read a startling newspaper report on fathers over 40. It claims that the older men become, the poorer the quality of the genetic material they transfer. If sperm cell fragmentation occurs, not only do the chances of miscarriage double – from 16.7 per cent for 30- to 35-year-old men to 32.7 per cent for men over 40, irrespective of the age of the mother – 'spelling mistakes' in the copying process can take place. For every man reproducing in his fifties, each will contribute to one in 200 extra births with serious health problems, including congenital abnormalities. This is the reason the maximum age for being a sperm donor was lowered from 45 to 40 in 2011. The article makes for disturbing reading. Are Emily's problems my fault?

We're having breakfast in the sun-filled lounge one Saturday morning when Anita casually says: 'Don't be alarmed, but I was reading on the Internet that babies not pointing or waving at 18 months – or responding to such gestures – is a red flag for autism.'

Even before the sentence is complete my arms are numb. A great weariness descends, as if I've been drugged. I stare at the food: poached eggs and muffins, with spinach and butter. A fruit salad: apple, banana, raspberries, blueberries, pear. Tea, coffee.

All is lost.

I don't know what to say or do. I have a sudden, irrational urge to tidy up. I leave the table, and walk around the room, hammering in all the floorboard nails that have raised in the warmer weather, while continuing the conversation in a sort of fugue state.

I have to get some air. I pull on my jacket and boots, grab my keys and fly down the stairs to the street. I run through Church Passage, then turn left onto Claremont Road. Is this what Emily has? Autism? I don't even know what autism is, not really. A lack of empathy? *Rain Man*? *The Curious Incident of the Dog in the Night-Time*?

The town seems to be filled with children and their parents. On the other side of the road I see a little girl walking, bobbing along – blonde curls, red Janis Joplin-style heart-shaped shades – talking to her dad.

All is lost.

I suddenly feel angry. The constant talk of 'Oh, she's just a late bloomer' is bullshit. I'm convinced of that now. Emily is autistic.

10

I Will

I'VE KNOWN FOR some time now that our experience of parenthood is diverging from the other NCT mums and dads. Emily is almost 18 months old, and, despite the breakthrough with her mobility, there is still little progress in any other area. She has no speech, nor any alternative form of communication.

It's a slender reed, but I cling to the fact she *is* interested in certain things, she is curious. She always has been. Her gazing at her reflection in the playmat's mirror as the Beach Boys played. How long ago and innocent that episode feels now. The whole happy era when we had no idea there was anything wrong with her development.

These are the days when rapid changes *must* occur, I tell myself. Two of the NCT mothers are pregnant again. That is unthinkable for us, with everything stalled at the moment. Out of all the parents in the group, it was Anita and I who had a baby that wasn't going to develop normally. These are the cards that have been dealt.

So deal.

Since the talk over breakfast, I notice references to autism everywhere. There's even a new BBC drama series, *The A Word*. But I refuse to Google the condition – almost as a badge of pride. I have never run to the Internet or textbooks with suspected medical problems. I can wait for a diagnosis – whatever that may be – from the professionals.

A few days later, alert to anything that might allay my fears, an incident at the nursery convinces me that Emily is not autistic. I arrive one afternoon to find her sitting on the floor with three or four other children, smiling. Suddenly, the boy next to her starts to cry. Big, bawling red-faced sobs. Emily drops the smile and turns to look at him. Slowly, a mournful expression of concern appears on her face, gradually deepening. An extraordinary transformation takes place: she seems to age five, 10, 20 years. Her eyes, shaded by her long lashes, are pools of deep empathy. Not the eyes of a child anymore, but those of a beautiful young woman. I stand mesmerised in the doorway, locked out of the scene. She puts her fingers to her lips … I'm certain that if she had more mobility she would have stood up and placed a reassuring hand on her poor screaming playmate's shoulder.

Abruptly, the boy stops crying, and Emily changes back into a child. The episode haunts me for the rest of the day. Surely an autistic kid couldn't do that, couldn't display so much empathy?

A Sunday morning. 10am. I wander into the airy, sun-bright living room. Anita is sitting on the sofa wearing pyjamas, knees pulled up to her chin, staring at the screen of her HP laptop. She says Emily isn't receiving the help she needs soon enough – the Portage and occupational therapists haven't been in touch yet.

'Everything's going too slow. The other kids are racing ahead.' There is deep grievance in her voice.

She starts crying. Long rivulets of tears curve down her cheeks. I pluck a tissue from the box on the dining table, and sit next to her on the sofa. Reaching around to massage her shoulders, I note they feel as hard as wood. I glance at the computer: a page on delayed development. I tell her softly that, up until now, her strength was keeping me strong. Anger flashes in her eyes. Don't criticise me for having my own doubts and fears, she says. But the truth is, I don't know what her doubts and fears are.

She leaps up and heads for the kitchen.

'They have her down at nursery as *Special*.' She spits the last word. 'Labelled already.'

I follow her into the other room, and start squeezing oranges. Now there is a hopeful note in her voice: 'I don't think Emily understands me, but when I say "window" or "bathroom", I feel like she leads me there.'

'When are they meant to understand?' I ask, knowing full well it's already.

'*Now*. The others find their shoes, or pretend to speak into a mobile phone ... And her hands – her motor skills aren't developing quickly enough.'

I watch my own hands pinch and squeeze the fruit as if they don't belong to me. Fear hums in my stomach.

'I just want to know what's wrong with her,' I say.

'Well, we may never know.'

I have a dream in which Emily is able to walk and talk. The three of us are on the sofa in the living room, Emily on Anita's lap, when she breaks free and says, 'Look, Mummy, I'm as quick as a hare!' Then she leaps behind the television and hangs upside down from the tangle of cables. I tell her off, something I've never had to do before. It's a strange, disturbing dream.

I wake at 6:30, and get her ready for nursery as usual. Perhaps unsurprisingly, she hasn't developed speech and mobility overnight.

Pointing the buggy down the steep incline that leads to the crèche, I notice there's something different about the line of sight ahead. All the young trees are out in fine white blossom.

'It's spring!' I shout, hoping Emily will hear, and somehow respond. I watch her eyes following the petals as they fall lightly through the air, or scurry across our path, driven by the breeze. They move frictionlessly along the road, everywhere. I run as fast as I can with the buggy, dodging reversing 4x4s setting out on the school run, and reach the gate at 8am sharp.

On the way back, I notice a poster in a charity shop window requesting donations for children with 'complex needs'. It shows Down's syndrome kids playing in a nursery setting. No one can say it, can they? *Special needs.*

The end of another day. Emily has drunk her milk without fuss, and compliantly allows me to balance her on my knee. She burps quietly, and I carry her over to our perch by the lounge window. A pale moon is beginning its arc above the spire of St Mark's. The sky is a flawless, cerulean blue. The road is empty save for the odd car.

'Car,' I say. 'Car!'

If only she could say just *one* word.

I sing her songs from the Beatles' *White Album*. 'Mother Nature's Son', 'Blackbird', 'I Will'. It strikes me it's no accident the working title for the record was *A Doll's House*, so many of the tunes sound like lullabies, or are about childhood. I begin a tremulous version of 'Good Night', the last song on the LP. Written by John for his son Julian; sung beautifully by Ringo.

I pick Emily up, walk slowly to the bathroom, and we sit on the edge of the tub. I clean her teeth with some effort: she doesn't like the brush anymore, just the taste of the toothpaste. Still singing the lugubrious melody – doing my best Ringo – I carry her into her bedroom. The blackout blind is drawn, the cot already prepared, sleeping bag ready, her soft-toy white rabbit in a corner. I gently lower her into the crib, place the dummy in her mouth. Then I thread her little fists through the armholes of the sleep-suit, pull up the zip, and fasten the clip at the top. She's looking up at me, eyes already closing, hugging the bunny, head turning sleepily from side to side. Sweet dreams, my darling girl. Sweet dreams.

11

Ascension Day

ANITA HAS APPLIED for a job at a school in Frankfurt. To celebrate, we head out to the Italian restaurant opposite the station, Emily in her buggy. We order spaghetti Bolognese and seafood linguine, which briefly ignites a flame of longing for strong sunlight and holiday evenings spent in trattorias with good red wine. *Sardinia* ... But then I remember Gran Canaria.

I cut up half my pasta for Emily, which she eats enthusiastically, then play peek-a-boo with her, using a small, soft yellow chick, the toy of the moment. Anita says that tomorrow our lives could change forever. She has a Skype interview with the school. I'm excited by this, but apprehensive. It's all moving too fast. I don't say anything.

On our return, she takes Emily out to the garden, to walk her. I watch them for a long time, from the high bathroom window; Emily small in her plum-coloured hoodie, Anita in her light summer coat. They make laps of the overgrown lawn, passing the bench by the dilapidated shed, which Emily clasps hold of, only to topple backwards into the matted grass. Anita picks her up, and they continue their circumnavigations. I try to imagine the three of us, living a new life in Germany …

The weakening afternoon sun warms my arms as I lean on the sash window. Above my head, a ladybird lands on the blind. *Paff.* Bathroom echo. I'm struck by how much Emily reminds me of photographs of my twin brother and I when we were little, the same thatch of tousled blond hair.

Suddenly, Anita notices me. She points to the window, encouraging Emily to follow her finger.

'Daddy!' She says. '*Da-da!*'

Emily doesn't look up.

The end of April. Emily is 18 months old, the last of the major date milestones before the age of two. She stands unassisted for the first time. It happens as Anita and I are walking her in the lounge. We let go, gingerly, and Emily stops moving, becomes completely still, like someone pausing in a game of statues. Then she falls back, into our waiting arms. We clap, and whoop our approval. *Bravo, Emily! Bravo!* Anita hugs her tightly. Do I imagine it, or is Emily's smile of pride and satisfaction – the one she tries to suppress (*who, me?*) – slightly more pronounced than usual, slightly harder for her to hide?

But she's still not walking.

Not walking at 18 months is when to worry.

The genetics appointment rolls around. We drive to the hospital, find the department, and sit outside the consultant's office, attempting to keep a restless Emily amused. The corridor is close and hot, and we only have a limited number of distractions for her.

Presently, Dr Hughes greets us, shows us into his room. He takes a seat behind his desk, a slim man in his late fifties, wearing a checked, short-sleeve shirt and slacks. Narrow face, cropped white hair, rimless, octagonal spectacles. I immediately notice his large, amused eyes. They transmit a sort of playful benevolence, which is encouraging. Perhaps he will be sympathetic to us, and to Emily. I hope so, as it's even hotter in his room than the corridor, and our daughter, sitting on Anita's lap, is already crying so loudly it's hard to hear what's being said.

'I'm here to put the pieces of the puzzle together,' Dr Hughes says, and continues with a few preliminary questions. When he learns I play music, he asks, 'Any band I would know?' I reply in the negative. He pauses, smiles.

'I only mention it because I once asked this of a patient, and the answer was Queen.'

An amusing anecdote to put us at our ease, a good sign.

Then he considers Emily.

'You're a pretty one … Hmm, not obvious from the face that she has any syndromes.'

Dr Hughes catches my alarmed look.

'A syndrome just means a collection of symptoms.'

He measures her head.

'Hmm … normal. The head's not helpful.'

He examines her hands and feet. I point out the large space after each of her big toes, which is similar to mine.

'My wife always laughs at my feet,' he says, solemnly.

Then he checks the inside of her mouth, lifting the NHS lanyard from around his neck to make Emily raise her chin. Her crying stops for a brief moment.

'Do you like my badge, pretty one?' he says. He is sensitive with her. 'Yes, her palette is rather high.'

Dr Hughes consults his notes for a moment, then speaks.

'Well, we have no clues to go on. Looking at her, I'm not convinced this is genetic. We need the other pieces of the jigsaw, and that will mean an MRI.'

Anita and I glance at each other nervously.

'We've decided not to go for the MRI until she's a bit older,' I say.

'Look, we can't say this is a brain damage scenario caused by lack of oxygen at birth unless we scan.'

Time stops.

Brain damage.

We haven't said anything about brain damage. I feel as if I'm back in the childhood dream, swimming at night in very cold, very deep water.

'We're really not that keen. At the moment,' I manage to say.

'If I could see something in the brain, damage from lack of oxygen, then we could see if it was maturing properly or not.'

I feel light-headed, sick.

Emily's crying is becoming louder and louder. Dr Hughes and I are now like two people trying to hold a conversation in the front row of a gig.

'I'm going to discuss this with my colleagues. But they will probably recommend an MRI. Otherwise it's scattergun tests across the genome, which could take years. Then you become a research project,' he smiles. 'Thousands of pounds, and I'm afraid we can't afford you.'

I mumble something non-committal.

'Do you want more kids?' he asks.

'Yes,' I reply, surprised at his question, and at how unequivocal my answer is.

'Good. Stick to it. That way you get more tests.'

Another smile.

Then the doctor takes photographs of Emily for the meeting with his fellow geneticists. She is inconsolable by now, howling and screaming, Anita doing her best to calm her.

'I'm going to recommend a blood test. A CGH microarray analysis. I'll be able to see from that if there are any deletions or duplications in the chromosome. And we go from there, OK?'

As we gather our belongings, I wonder if I should mention autism, but the moment passes. Instead, I ask if he thinks my age could be a reason for Emily's problems. He dismisses the idea: 'Don't blame yourself. We did factor it in once, but the dad was 75.'

It's a minor relief.

He shows us politely out of his office.

In the car park, the hot afternoon burns on. I can't seem to think coherently anymore. We still haven't resolved whether or not to risk the MRI. It's starting to feel inevitable.

*

It's one of those fresh, blue mornings in May, the sun already high at 8:30am, the air damp and full of mingling scents. Soil, petrol, pollen.

Changes are occurring. Emily squirms and wriggles as if there is new energy within her. Her will is becoming stronger. She wants to walk all the time, held by her fingertips, of course, otherwise she would keel over. We charge through the flat, avoiding the nails. And she can, with much difficulty, raise herself onto four points. The breakthrough last month wasn't a fluke. The weight-bearing exercises have given her more strength in the shoulder muscle girdle. She soon collapses, her tiny frog-like legs kicking, back arched, pounding the mat in frustration – thwarted again – but this would have been unthinkable eight weeks ago. In this position she can rotate on her belly, reach out to toys.

Is it happening at last? The thing I wish for day and night? With the acceleration of May all around, I think – I hope – it might be.

It's happening. When I pick up Emily from nursery in the afternoon, the staff are eager to tell me about her latest achievements. The key worker, kneeling on the floor, attempting to put the plum-coloured cardigan back onto a wriggling Emily, looks up at me earnestly.

'She really wants to walk, sir.'

Yes. Yes, she does, I agree. Then she informs me how much Emily enjoyed playing with some Hundreds and Thousands earlier, and points to a Tupperware box on a shelf, marked 'Emily'. I feel a stab of pain that she has her own special box, but it passes.

'We keep all her sensory stuff in there,' she says.

As I carry Emily away, I hear the key worker say to another

staff member, 'She's coming on in leaps and bounds, that one,' and I no longer have any doubts that they're all behind her, urging her on, willing her to succeed. It moves me deeply.

I'm fired up by the idea of living abroad, yet the fear is immense, waking me at 3am with a feeling that something dreadful has happened. The decision is a terrible mistake, and will have to be reversed. What if the project is a disaster and we have to return, bridges burned? Would I get my old gigs – residencies that have taken years to establish – back? Someone will take my place. But after a few moments these anxieties subside, and I see the many benefits, especially for Emily. The artistic advantages, too. With a lower cost of living, I could finally be free to write. I think loftily of Wordsworth and Coleridge in Göttingen. Bowie in Berlin. A new career in a new town. Just for a couple of years ...

Emily has been crawling. Only a few paces, then she seems to forget how to do it, and collapses onto her belly. Anita and I look on in amazement. Only days earlier, at the crèche, I watched with the usual envy as one of her playmates crawled. He couldn't have been more than ten months old, and had clearly only just learned this new skill. He elbowed his way jerkily across the floor, like someone swimming, but practising all the strokes at once – front crawl, breaststroke, butterfly. Now I'm gripped by the conviction that Emily will soon be able to move like him.

One morning in late May, the Portage home visitor comes to

the flat. The woman explains to us how the therapy acquired its name (a town in America where the techniques were pioneered) and how it works. Portage is an intervention that teaches children with 'additional needs' new skills via the use of prompts, tasks and rewards. She has brought a large container of sensory toys with her, and some useful information. Apparently, children develop strength from the inside out: core stability begets coarse motor skills, which beget fine motor skills. Moreover, the weight-bearing action of crawling sends stimuli to the brain, which unlocks the desire to learn. The physical engenders the mental.

Later, in the afternoon, a speech and language therapist visits. The session starts well, but she asks so many questions about my interaction with Emily that, after a while, I begin to feel uncomfortable.

'How do you play with her?'

'I don't know, I just make it up as I go along!'

'How do you feel about that?'

Anita looks at me; raises an eyebrow.

The therapist suggests filming me as I play with Emily. I mess around on the playmat with her for a while, then throw a ball in the air to make her laugh. The woman asks more questions. Maybe I'm just tired from the morning, but I can't find the answers, and feel flustered, like a schoolboy.

As she's summing up, she casually says, 'Of course, Emily may never speak.'

At first, I think I've misheard her. I catch Anita, sitting at the dining table, visibly flinch.

After the therapist has left, I erupt with anger. How could

she say that in front of two desperately worried parents? *May never speak?* I've never heard of a child that couldn't speak. Then something silences me. During my outburst, Anita has been checking her phone. An email offering her the job in Germany has arrived.

Momentous days follow. The move to Frankfurt is going ahead. Anita makes the final arrangements with the school – an employment contract (including a 3,000-euro relocation fee) has been verbally agreed. Every hour, my mind reels with the logistics of the operation: parking permits for the removal lorry, haulage costs, insurances, apartments, nursery places, *work* ... But we are going, in August, it seems. So soon.

And Emily is crawling properly, at last. Her first few tentative paces have become, in the space of a week, ever-more confident expeditions across the playmat to locate a toy. This is unmistakable progress. Finally crawling, at 18-and-a-half months. Watching her, Anita and I can't stop smiling. We high-five, stare, *gawp* at our daughter.

*

May slips into June. Emily's progress is rapid, dazzling. She can crawl all the way to the kitchen, and change orientation at will on the playmat to investigate something that has caught her interest. She is able to raise herself up on the low radiator beneath the lounge window, and, with enormous effort – limbs trembling – stand upright, hands clasped on the sill. Anita's eyes become misty when she speaks of Jane, whom she rightly considers the catalyst for Emily's new mobility.

Yesterday, when I reported the latest developments to the nursery key worker, I feared she was going to burst into tears, such was the rapt, wide-eyed intensity of her stare. It feels as if everyone's faith in our daughter is finally being redeemed.

I was unprepared for this sudden leap; accustomed to her being stuck, trapped – an eight-month-old in an 18-month-old body. Often, I can't believe what I'm seeing. It just looks so unusual to see Emily move around like this. And perhaps it feels strange for her, too, because she now has some agency of her own.

Firsts occur almost every day now. She can raise herself to a standing position in the cot with both hands. Sometimes, when I pass her room, I catch a glimpse of two little fists gripping the bars, like a prisoner, and I remember Anita's remark, back in November – *Won't it be great when we find her in the morning, doing this on her own?* – and how much I doubted it would ever happen. We are in a constant state of euphoria. One morning, I put a *Supremes Best Of* on the stereo before feeding Emily breakfast. Anita comes into the room, edges up the volume to 'Love Is Like An Itching In My Heart', and dances our daughter around, holding her high above her head. Emily screams with delight, the happiest of smiles on her face.

The follow-up appointment with the consultant paediatrician, Dr McNally, arrives. We visit him at the hospital this time. He greets us with smiles in a small, airless room, wearing a blue NHS shirt and slacks. Only a pair of Prince of Wales checked socks visible above his slip-ons echoes the subtly dandified appearance from last December. He transmits more sympathy during this second meeting (or maybe we are less defensive), asks us if we're all right, as parents. Are we coping? We tell him that it's been a tough six months, but we have some good news: Emily is crawling, at last.

He performs a few routine tests, makes some notes.

'She is still very delayed,' he announces, 'but I'm pleased with her progress. When I first saw her, I was worried. She was severe.'

He asks if we've seen Dr Hughes yet, the geneticist. I say we have, and he was insistent on the MRI.

McNally sits motionless in his chair, gold pen in hand.

'Only with an MRI can we find out exactly what's wrong.'

I decide to ask him one of the questions that has been consuming me for some time: 'Does there actually have to *be* anything wrong? A *reason* for the delay?'

'No,' he replies, 'in 50 per cent of the cases there is no reason.' He registers the relief on our faces, then continues, 'But I'm happy not to risk the MRI for the time being, if you are worried.'

The room seems to be getting hotter and hotter. Emily, sitting on Anita's knee, is recreating the scene from Dr Hughes's office. Her crying is now so loud and persistent we can barely hear ourselves speak.

Taking a deep breath, I ask about brain damage. He considers Emily once more.

'It doesn't look like brain damage … she's not stiff. Is she showing what she wants? Does she get angry?'

Can he *hear* Emily? I wonder.

'Yes, yes she does. Could it be autism?'

'We can't rule that out.'

I feel my chest tighten. I'm unable to comprehend we're even talking about this.

'At aged four she could be two, at ten she could be eight,' he continues, 'I'm not going to say everything is all right.' And I remember this phrase from the first meeting, the awful rush of cortisone it produced in my stomach. 'Look,' he says, 'keep your hopes up. I'm very pleased with her progress.'

'But we're not out of the woods, right?' I ask.

Just at that moment, McNally leans forward, and stares intently at Emily. She has stopped crying momentarily, placated by a rice cake. What has he seen? Some behavioural tic, or physical sign? He resembles a zoologist studying a very rare insect, a look of entomological absorption on his face.

I don't ask what has caught his attention, but later, at home, I will wish I had. The session is over.

'Come back again in six months,' he says.

Then: 'Are you going anywhere over the summer?'

Anita and I look at each other nervously.

'Ah, travelling, maybe ...' I say.

The doctor nods.

Outside, in the car park, my head is spinning. I can't operate the ticket machine; can't get the ends of the child seat belt to connect properly. Attempting to strap Emily in, stooped and twisted and trying not to accidentally knock her head as she screams and howls, I lose my temper. Anita asks me what's wrong. Em's crying is *boiling my piss*, that's what's fucking well wrong, I say.

I sit in the back as the car moves off, my face stinging with shame. I wasn't prepared for how deeply the appointment would affect me. A sense of impotence, failure – that I can't control what is happening – has me in its grip. I notice Anita's quietly concerned expression in the rear-view. She takes one hand off the wheel, and reaches round behind her seat to gently stroke my ankle.

'I'm just frustrated that there are no answers,' I finally manage to say, 'that we don't know how it's going to turn out.'

'That's life though, isn't it?' Anita says, with perfect logic. 'We don't know how it turns out.'

*

Events are moving so fast it is hard to keep pace. The relocation – or 'emigration', as several friends have called it – is a mere three-and-a-half weeks away. We've handed in our notice on the flat – which is frightening, as we don't yet have a place to live in Germany. An apartment has been located, but we're still waiting to hear back from the landlord, who is choosing between us and another couple. If the flat falls through, we must start looking again, and the timeframe to do that is worryingly tight. Meanwhile, the packing boxes from the removal company have arrived. They stand unassembled in the hall, in great drifts, a delightful new play area for Emily. I make trips to charity shops with old clothes, hand-me-down toys.

Happily, though, Emily's physical development is showing no signs of slowing down. She can crawl with ease now, push the First-Steps baby walker across the lounge, move about while being held only around her waist. She is becoming an adept mountaineer on the sofa, too; judging heights, distances, foot and hand holds, which areas will give her leverage, which will slip away. And she has finally moved upstairs at the nursery, joining her mobile contemporaries – a milestone.

I break the news to Laura that we're moving to Germany. I find I have to control the emotion in my voice when I thank her for everything they have done. I feel nothing but guilt for the way I doubted them. But maybe all parents in our situation are equally paranoid. I can't be sure, we don't know any.

On a warm day in July, Emily takes her first unassisted steps. Three paces only, but they may as well be three paces on water. Or the moon. I watch from high above in the mezzanine as Anita conducts the experiment on the playmat. We roar and clap as if we were in a theatre. *You did it! We're so proud of you!* At last – she can walk.

All that remains now is for her brain to be developing normally.

*

One evening in the lounge, Emily and I watch a spectacular summer thunderstorm. I hold her up to the window as the rain pounds the road below, the tarmac slick and undulating, the gutters running with twigs and leaf debris. Beneath an orange streetlight, it looks as if a swarm of wasps is thrashing angrily around and around. She's in fits of laughter, strikes her open palms on my chest; looks up at me with the broadest smile. I tell her jokingly it was me who made it rain, with a special machine called a Cloudbuster, and I wonder how she would she respond if she could speak.

No you didn't, Daddy! Don't be silly!

But I don't know how she would respond, not really, for she has no words yet. And, of course, as we all know, *Emily may never speak.*

Eight am. The last day before the move. I sit on the rusting fire escape with a cup of coffee, the sun hot on my neck, watching the cobwebs sparkle, trying to keep calm. We have finally secured an apartment in a quiet suburb of Frankfurt, but there is still much to organise. Later, I sell the Renault for cash, to a young teacher from East Cheam, getting back a fraction of what I paid for it. I cancel all upcoming hospital appointments, including the genetics blood test, and one for an MRI, which the NHS generated by mistake. We take a final walk by the river, which on this hot summer's day is a rich, unctuous green, like posh olive oil. Then we swelter, packing last boxes, Emily crawling around in only her nappy.

Later still, we hold a barbecue in the garden for friends, family, and the NCTs. Our downstairs neighbours, Anna and Roberto, are here, too. If they think we're mad, moving abroad so suddenly, they don't show it.

It's dusk by the time I've hefted the last bags of empty beer bottles into the recycling, made the final journey upstairs with leftovers, ready to be cling-filmed for the fridge. I place the smouldering barbecue in the centre of the garden with the lid open. Then Anita and I sit high up on the fire escape with glasses of wine, watching the embers glow, talking about the days to come. She and Emily will go on ahead to her parents in Germany, while I oversee the removal here.

The sun is sinking behind the houses, casting chimney

pots in a muted yellow light. Charcoal shapes – swifts – shoot upwards. I point out the strange, flattened cedar, now an inscrutable silhouette in the middle distance. I tell Anita that I once made up a story for Emily about this tree, how a giant was walking towards Richmond one day, became tired, and sat down on it to rest awhile. Soon, I say, she will be able to tell us stories of her own.

I propose a toast: Here's to the future, and to Emily.

Emily's future.

Part II

*Age 22 months to two-
and-a-half years*

12

The Thoughts Of Mary Jane

Frankfurt, September 2016

SIX WEEKS LATER. We live on the first floor of a refurbished 1950s block, above an *Optiker*. The flat – sorry, the *apartment* – is enormous. Emily's room is three times the size of her previous one, dwarfing the IKEA cot we've brought with us from England. Everything – the doors, the windows – seems to fit, to work, unlike the old Heath Robinson Bond flat in Surbiton. What's more, everything about the apartment *feels* different, exotic. In the mornings, the echoing, green faux-marble stairwell smells of cigarette smoke and aftershave, which I don't find irritating, because it is European cigarette smoke, and European aftershave. The light switches and *Klingel* are the original dark brown Bakelite fittings, like props from a Fritz Lang film.

We have a balcony, too, with a view of the new neighbourhood; which is quiet, somnambulant, even, at times. Our street is cobbled, with *fin-de-siècle* gas lamps. Sometimes, in the evenings, I imagine I can hear horse-drawn carriages below, the sound of hooves. And every 15 minutes: the bells. Not the pastoral melody of English bells, but the ringing one hears in an arthouse movie – a Czech or Viennese square. We are close to an enormous Catholic church, visible from the kitchen window, partially hidden behind a tall Norwegian spruce. I find it odd, yet fitting, that we should look out onto a church spire once again.

This will be a real home for Emily, I think to myself each day, as I unpack the last of the boxes. Her lion print is already up on the wall in her room. In the spacious kitchen, the new AEG fridge will soon be covered with her kindergarten artwork, which I'm confident she will have the skills to produce before long. And the wide corridor which links each room – smoothly laminated, and nail-free – offers her much more space to practise her newfound mobility.

Every day I am borne up on a wave of nervous energy. I haven't read a single newspaper or watched any television. It's cleansing, in a strange way. And it still feels odd to reach into my left-hand jeans pocket and not find my Oyster card.

There are two small music venues, where I'm hoping to find work. Although, worryingly, there only seem to be posters for tribute bands on their walls. Custard Pie (Led Zeppelin), Marley's Ghost (self-explanatory), and my favourite – Dire Strats. I'm not brave enough to order a glass of *Pilsner*, let alone ask for a gig in either of these places yet, so I begin practising my German in the nearby *Bäkerei*. '*Ich hätte gerne eine Latte, bitte*,' – I would like a latte, please – to small, embarrassed smiles from the girls behind the counter.

At the weekends, Anita and I motor into central Frankfurt in our new (second-hand) VW Polo, Emily in the back. Through the open windows come continental smells of coffee, bread. I'm thrilled by the torrent of new sights flashing by in the Indian summer sunshine, although to Anita they will seem familiar, homely. A market selling strawberries so red and glossy they look like fakes; the broad, boat-strewn River Main; the domed spire of the Liebfrauenkirche reflecting the light on Liebfrauenberg. Everywhere there is something of interest: tall, turn-of-the-century houses – grand villas with cream, pink or peach facades. Carved Art Nouveau faces glimpsed high up on ornate cornicing. Newer, 1970s concrete builds, with chocolate-brown tiled roofs and balconies. Old fifties shop signs, with cursive neon fonts. A painted figure of the Virgin Mary on the corner of a *Gasthaus*. Mysterious Catholic chalk symbols and numbers by apartment doors. And everyone, it seems, has a bicycle; they glide past continually, some with balsa-wood grocery baskets, others towing child trailers.

I study the people on the streets. They seem to have created a mandate to enjoy life, not merely grind themselves into the dirt working, as everyone does in London. They strike me as eminently sane – shopping leisurely for groceries, or whizzing past on bikes, laughing. It is as if they know the secret of life. And it is this life, in a small town in Germany, with a summer winding down, that I want for my family.

Anita has begun the slow process of registering Emily with a new paediatrician and therapists. She has also started full-time at the school, which leaves me looking after our daughter. Until we find day care – the kindergartens are fully booked, and *Tagesmütter* (childminders) seem to be non-existent – this is my current occupation. Each morning, I roam the streets, Emily in the buggy, the strong late-September sun on our faces. Temperatures are still in the thirties, and the stench from the Orange *Stadt* refuse trucks is sweet. There is dust on my boots; and my thumbs, from hours gripping the pushchair handles, have turned brown.

When the afternoons become too muggy, we go off-road, and look for some green space.

During these walks, I have a much-loved artist on the iPod: Nick Drake. Although a more English singer-songwriter would be hard to imagine, Drake's breathy, classical voice and agile, hypnotic guitar figures somehow complement this peaceful part of Germany. Back in the eighties, the only Nick Drake record I owned was a *Best Of*. I'd read his name in the music papers, dropped by another Nick – Nick Laird-Clowes, who, with his band the Dream Academy, had just released the panoramic single 'Life In A Northern Town'. One day, without knowing what the other Nick sounded like, not even a note, I decided to buy the *Best Of* from the local record shop. I was 16, and it was 1985. The black-and-white cover image was a headshot of a serious-looking young man, with a heavy, sensitive lower lip, his features framed by long, dark hair, eyes obscured by the title: *Heaven in a Wild Flower: An Exploration of Nick Drake*. This was exciting. As a serious, long-haired young man myself, a poet and songwriter, too (and an A-level English student who still lived at home with his mum), I knew 'heaven in a wild flower' was a line from Blake's 'Auguries Of Innocence'. It alluded to an idea I was passionately interested in at the time: Pantheism, the idea of the holy in nature. I decided to take the risk, and put my hand in my pocket.

On the bus back, I read the sleeve notes. They revealed details of Drake's short, troubled life. Born to upper-middle-class parents in 1948, shy, sensitive Nick was educated at Marlborough, then later Cambridge, where he dropped out to make a trilogy of critically favoured but poor-selling albums. Beset by mental health issues, and considering himself a failure, he retreated to the family home, where he began contemplating a new career in either the army or computers. He died, unknown to the general public, aged 26, from an accidental (some say deliberate) overdose of antidepressants.

Expecting bleak music, when I got home and listened to Heaven in a Wild Flower I was surprised to find songs that were light, optimistic. Yes, there was melancholy, and some flashes of darkness, but in his simple lyrics with their motifs borrowed from the French symbolists – sun, moon, rain, trees – there was much to enjoy. The standout song, for me, was 'River Man', in languid, jazzy 5/4, with Delius-like strings that conjured up a June day in the English countryside: high clouds inching imperceptibly across a deep blue sky, bees and butterflies in the glades, and the sound of a whispering river, coming and going.

It is this song I play the most on these wanderings, along with another from *Heaven in a Wild Flower*, 'The Thoughts Of Mary Jane'. In the lyric, Drake is trying to imagine what is in the mind of a strange girl, who, he says, is on a journey to the stars. It makes me think of Emily.

One towering Indian summer afternoon, I find myself pushing the buggy through a wood that leads to a nearby playground. I put the brake on, and crouch down. Cabbage whites flip-flop in the deep green shade of vegetation around us. I adjust Emily's white sun-bonnet, offer her the water cup. She takes a sip; big thirsty eyes wide open, looking straight ahead. We are on a small bridge over a stream. Emily gazes at the water's ever-changing patterns, the glittering points of smashed light that seem to hover just above the surface. Is she seeing the holy in nature? Heaven in a wild river? I wish I could tune into her thoughts, the thoughts of Mary Jane.

'We're in *Germany* ...' I whisper. 'Will you remember?'

She stares at the black water as it bubbles over the rocks on the streambed, following the ripples with her blue-grey eyes, immersed in her solitude.

One evening towards the end of September, sitting on the balcony with Anita drinking wine – watching the flares of shooting stars overhead – she says a doctor asked if Emily had been deprived of oxygen at birth. I experience that old, cold feeling in the pit of my stomach. The spectre of her delayed development still haunts me, but in the past month-and-a-half the thought has become less intrusive. Her mobility continues to improve; she can run now – albeit a very unsteady, chaotic type of running. She can switch from walking to crawling, and turn with ease. The only thing she can't do yet is raise herself from a sitting position to a stand. She seems so much happier with her new freedom, and all the space in which to express it. She cries much less.

But the physiotherapist made comments, too, according to Anita. He said Emily is not aware of him, or doesn't seem to need to interact with him when she plays. I cleave to the hope that this is because of her glue ear – she is still partially deaf. We have a hospital appointment soon for a procedure to remove the fluid. I'm trying to quell my fears; focus on what she *can* do rather than what she cannot.

I say nothing; just stare into the cool, blue *Himmel* above, waiting for another soundless comet to appear.

A recent memory returns. It's hard to be sure, but last Sunday, eating breakfast in the lounge with Emily, she looked at Anita and said, *Ma-ma*.

Mama?

Then, later, directed towards me: *Ba-Ba-Ba-Ba* ...

Maybe the paradiddle worked: *Mum-my, Dad-dy, Mum-my, Dad-dy.*

Could this be the start? I'm hoping so much it hurts.

As the dusk gathers, and shapes soften, Anita closes her eyes. I wonder if she's seen a shooting star and is wishing upon it. After she's gone to bed, I sit nursing the last of the wine in the warm European night, hoping to see another. But none appears. I had my wish ready: please, just let our child be normal.

*

At the start of October, with much luck and pulling-of-strings, we find a childminder. A friendly Estonian woman who lives in an apartment on a nearby *Straße*, reached by climbing five flights of rickety wooden stairs. Today is Emily's first day.

It's 7am, and we're in our kitchen, getting ready. Through the open window comes the smell of car tyre-y air; sounds of metal shutters being raised, children laughing and shouting on their way to *Schule*. Early morning in a sleepy German suburb. I sit Emily in her new moulded plastic high chair, put 'grippy' socks on her feet (the laminated floors are slippery and her balance is still off), a pair of *Hausschuhe* – indoor shoes – for warmth, and we're all set for breakfast. I sing for her as the spoon goes in. This morning's tune: David Bowie's 'The Prettiest Star'.

I've been thinking about her response to music. Everyone comments on it. She seems to latch onto a song far more readily than speech. Sometimes, when I speak to her, she sends me a puzzled, unsure look (if she's in the mood for eye contact), and I can see her struggling to decipher what I mean, as if I've given her a quadratic equation to solve. Other times, her expression is haughty, disdainful: *why are you constantly making that strange noise?* With music, it's different. There are definite signs of recognition from her when I play the opening phrases of 'Wish You Were Here' on the acoustic guitar. Not the main riff that sounds, on the record, as if it's coming out of a transistor radio, but the lonely, sorrowing lead part above it. She stops what she's doing and smiles. Once I discover this, I play it for her every day. She giggles sometimes when I fret the high-pitched double-note lick that appears about halfway through the intro. It *does* sound rather funny, or at least incongruous, when I think about it. Is this why she laughs?

I've written a song for her that elicits a similar reaction. I say 'song', it's just her name, really. It has a somewhat ambiguous key centre.

Em – i – ly (cha, cha, cha)
Em – i – ly (cha, cha, cha)
Etc.

And sometimes I add, to the same melody:

We love you,
Yes we do!

It's no more than a ditty, but she grins when I sing it, so I add it to the setlist.

Rhythmically, it's extremely versatile. I always clap along – fours or eighth notes, accents – her holding onto my wrists. The rhythm transfers to her, and often it feels as if she's in time, operating my hands, not the other way round.

I clear away the breakfast, and prepare Emily for her big day.

There's a discreet fringe of yellow leaves as I gun the buggy down the steep cut beside the church that leads to the childminder's. The air is cool, confirming the approach of autumn. Emily flaps her hands in delight at every passing cyclist, dog or pedestrian. When I've hefted her up the five flights, and ring the *Klingel* to the apartment, she gives me the smile, the one everyone waits to see; that grin of sheer delight – and my heart soars.

*

It's five days since the procedure to remove Emily's ear fluid. Her hearing seems to have improved dramatically. The sounds she makes are different; she responds to music more rapidly; doesn't burst into tears if a saucepan lid happens to clatter to the floor. I wince when I think of her constant crying in Gran Canaria – maybe the obstruction amplified a frequency that caused her actual physical pain. The plane journey must have been hell. Now she charges around the apartment, laughing jubilantly.

The day before Emily's second birthday, my mother and her partner, Ian, visit from England. We book a nearby Greek restaurant. It's cosy and inviting, with low wooden beams, thick white stone walls, candles, and copper jugs of wine next to gratis shots of ouzo on the tables. I sit beside Emily, feeding her the generously large, golden chips that come with the mixed grill. After each one, she looks up at me with that broad, joyful, tiny-toothed grin; and in the burnished glow from the candles, and with the ouzo's flame taking hold, my heart is more full of love than I imagined it could ever be.

The next day, Emily is two. And constipated. I blame the chips, personally. She lies on her front, legs outstretched, straining and uttering fearful cries. A trip to the nearby *Apotheke* for laxatives soon solves the problem, and she is ready for her party.

Anita has put up balloons and bunting. *Two Today!* The in-laws arrive with Emily's cousins, and a wonderful present: a Wendy house with a ball pond. I feel a surge of pride for Emily as she sits at the head of the table, the candles on her cake lit, all of us singing for her. My mum and Ian, the cousins, everybody celebrating her second year of life: *Happy Birthday, dear Emily, Happy Birthday to you!* I film the scene on my phone, trying to keep to the back of my mind that she looks confused, and is dribbling. I have a strong urge to press 'stop' and wipe the spittle from her chin. But I don't; I join in with the others. In this joyous, universal moment – a child's birthday party – the massed voices reassure me that she's going to be all right. Yes, dear Emily is going to be all right.

13

Waterfront

WHAT MAKES US human? Language? Concepts? Relating to others? These are questions that have been vexing me recently, because, as October becomes November, I'm becoming increasingly bleak about Emily's development. Her unexpected triumph back in the summer – crawling and walking within the space of a few weeks, and the immense project of relocating to a foreign country – has blindsided me. While her physical accomplishments are undeniable, her mental development seems to be static. Her cognition, her basic comprehension of situations appears to be practically zero. What brain-related activities can she do now that she couldn't a year ago? Complete a jigsaw? Draw a picture? Say even a simple word? Her only sounds are her rare vocalisms. Sometimes, she turns her head, looks away into the distance, and tests these utterances quietly, as if remembering something from a dream, while moving her hands in odd ways, her old Shirley Bassey shapes.

Moreover, perhaps I imagine it, but since she learned to walk she seems to interact with us less, make less eye contact. Peek-a-boo has vanished. She appears perfectly content to wander unsteadily and aimlessly from room to room, ignoring us when we call her name, or bashing a plastic shaker for what seems like hours on a marble windowsill.

When Anita returns from physiotherapy with Emily one afternoon, I mention my concerns. She says she stops breathing when anyone says our daughter isn't developing like other children.

'Did someone say something?' I ask.

'No,' she says, suddenly flustered. Her face reddens, and her eyes brim with tears.

Someone *did* say something.

That night, awake in the small hours, I'm assailed by dreadful thoughts. What if Emily really is intellectually disabled? The idea of raising such a child terrifies me. Soiling your nappy is fine when you're two, but not when you're 12, or 22, or 52. Who will change her nappy then, when Anita and I are no longer around? I'm gripped by fear, and a feeling of being utterly out of my depth; a conviction that, despite my age and supposed life experience, I'm not equipped to deal with any of this. Emily is going to have an awful life. *We*, as parents, are going to have an awful life. And this last, selfish, base thought lingers shamefully until the mercy of sleep finally comes. Yet when morning arrives – and I find Emily standing in her cot, smiling, ready for the day ahead – her sheer delight at being alive erases the night's terrors.

For the time being.

It's later the following week that events take a darker turn. I'm in the living room – a cold, damp November evening setting in – watching Emily shamble around happily, when I decide to Google 'odd hand movements in toddlers'.

A page of autism links appears.

I click on the first one.

An article from a US website fills the screen, the text divided into what an autistic child 'might' or 'might not' do.

They might: have unusual body or hand movements; play with toys in an odd way, or not at all; exhibit unusual sensory sensitivities. *They might not*: respond to their name; speak by 12 to 14 months; have good eye contact; point at objects or point to request something; attempt to gain the attention of other people; look when you direct their attention …

By the time Anita arrives home from work I'm in a state of complete panic. Emily has almost all the classic early warning signs of autism, 'a devastating neurological condition', according to the piece, which, for the so-called 'low- functioning' sufferers, can lead to a lifetime in care.

I remember now the child pointing at the car in Surbiton, and wondering why Emily had never done this. With a jolt, I remember Laura and Jane's concerns about eye contact. Then, with a burning in my stomach, I remember the only underlined words in Dr McNally's report last December: '*She did not have good eye contact with me at all in the clinic.*' Did they suspect autism all along? And, if so, why the hell didn't they say anything? Reading further, I discover that some autistic children never learn to speak, are 'nonverbal'. So that's why the speech therapist said what she said.

She knew.

Then I read about something called 'the triad of impairment'. It's here the link between pointing – what I considered a fairly important motor skill, but not as crucial as crawling or walking – and eye contact, which I thought was non-essential (and if poor, maybe something to do with shyness), becomes clear. Autistic children have three main areas of impairment: verbal and nonverbal communication, imaginative play, and social interaction. Take 'gaze shifts', for example. A normal child, playing with a toy, finding it delightful, looks to his parents to share his happiness, then returns to the toy. This is a gaze shift, apparently. Emily has never done this. And 'social referencing' – a child, engaged in an activity, tries to read his mother's face for approval. If she is smiling, he will carry on; if frowning, he might stop. Emily has never done this. Going further – 'joint attention'. This is when a child wants to share something using 'proto-declarative' pointing – at a car, say, to gain his mum's attention (*Ka!*). A toddler urgently wants to share his world with a grown-up. When both are looking at the car, this is joint attention. Emily has never …

I read on in a frenzy. Article after article. One mother describes her 27-month-old autistic son. It could be Emily. 'He refuses to look me in the eye for long, or listen to stories; he babbles but nothing clear. He was late walking and is still very clumsy. He makes spit puddles and cannot follow any directions …'

One newspaper piece asserts that autism can be detected by an fMRI, a functional MRI brain scan. A conviction is overturned in seconds: this is what Emily must have, and we need to bury our fears about the general anaesthetic. Most importantly, all the articles insist that early intervention is key. Two pieces state that the rapid introduction of autism therapies can cut symptoms in later life by *half*. This, one author expands, is because most of the brain connections needed for the development of complex social behaviours are established in the first three years. Treatment needs to start when the 'learning machinery is constantly switched on' – before mature brain circuitry is established.

After half an hour, I stop. I cannot read any further. I feel nauseous. Why wasn't I brave enough to confront this before, back in April, when Anita brought up lack of pointing as a possible 'red flag' for autism? Because I was always so proud of not running to the Internet for medical information, that's why. We could be putting treatment in place for Emily right now. I'm seized by a sickening urge to take action *immediately*.

I scoop up Emily, who has been throwing a small plastic football on the floor for the past 30 minutes, and walk to the kitchen. I find Anita opening bills and making coffee. I start preparing dinner, but can't keep the stress out of my actions, bashing drawers and cursing, until she asks what's wrong.

I tell her about my afternoon's reading, blurt it all out. The warning signs, the half-digested jargon. 'Gaze shifts', 'joint attention', 'the triad of impairment'. The urgent need for an fMRI. The urgent need to take action *now*.

'This is a countdown,' I say, 'a race against time to … save Emily's life.' The words sound ridiculous, insane even, as they leave my mouth, but I believe them nonetheless.

Anita looks sceptical.

'If that sounds melodramatic,' I continue, 'consider this: what happens now may impact everything that takes place in her life; every friendship, relationship, job. Everything. Her entire future is at stake.'

There's antagonism between us now.

'Look,' says Anita, pointing at Emily, 'she's looking straight at you. Giving you eye contact.'

I'm holding Emily over my shoulder while I stir a saucepan with my free hand. She's slapping my chin and laughing.

Anita asks: 'Are you going to call her autistic in front of people?'

'Yes,' I reply, 'if diagnosed. Rather that than they think she's a *half-wit*.'

Something in Anita's expression worries me, something like contempt.

We have an appointment with a neurologist tomorrow at one of the most renowned children's hospitals in Germany, their Great Ormond Street. We need to brace ourselves for the worst, I say.

Emily wakes up crying in the middle of the night. I go to her room, replace the dummy, settle her, but when I return I find I can't sleep. My mind is roiling with the old fears, and new, awful, bitter thoughts. All those dreams I had for her: ballet lessons and books, learning a musical instrument, marriage and a career – all that is smashed to pieces now. In the bin. A normal path through life is being denied her. The only thing that remains is damage limitation, via the therapies that we must set in motion right away.

The next day, we drive to the hospital, Emily in the back,

crossing the Main, its far banks veiled in river mist. In the car park, I carry my daughter through freezing sleet to reception. Snow is on the way.

The white buildings are low, modern, and in striking contrast to a British hospital, almost completely devoid of people. In the spacious waiting room is a play area with an impressively large, solid pine boat. I take Emily to the wheelhouse and the prow. I watch her interact with two other children. She smiles at an older boy, who sniggers at her innocent friendliness.

After a short wait, the neurologist, Dr Maier – a cheerful woman in her early forties, well-dressed in matching purples – welcomes us into her office. I look around the bright, clean space, so different to its British equivalent. It speaks of money and efficiency, more like a private healthcare setting than a public one. We're in the right place at last, I think to myself.

Dr Maier seems sympathetic, and agrees to speak in English as best she can.

'So,' she begins, 'are you here because you're worried, or because a doctor has said they're worried?'

Oh no.

She isn't aware of Emily's medical history. We have to start from the beginning. Within minutes everyone is talking over each other in two languages, attempting to establish the facts. I sit red-faced with self-loathing, yet knowing I have to say as much as I can about Emily's behaviour. It transpires we could have sent the hospital our discharge reports from the consultant paediatrician and Harefield House. Instead, the neurologist only has a questionnaire that we completed. It was all they asked for.

When everyone has calmed down, Dr Maier says, 'I didn't realise your daughter was so severe.'

Emily's problems are discussed one by one. Anita, standing in the centre of the room, holding Emily up by her hands, seems weary, as if she has a great weight on her shoulders. The doctor keeps using the word 'retarded'.

'Delayed,' corrects Anita.

Then I mention autism.

'Do you think we should get Emily screened for it?' I ask.

'Yes, I do,' Dr Maier says.

A shockwave goes through me. I was expecting the usual evasions. Before long, we're talking freely about the condition. Dr Maier is keen to emphasise the achievements of the higher-functioning individuals. But her tone soon begins to grate.

'Many autistic people can speak, and are highly intelligent,' she says brightly, at one point.

'Yes,' says Anita, 'I know,' staring distractedly at Emily, all her teaching experience showing in her face.

For a moment I wonder if we *are* in the right place. The paperwork was mishandled – not a good start. But the neurologist is already suggesting an autism assessment with a developmental psychologist, in January. And an immediate genetics investigation: the blood test, the CGH micro-array analysis that Dr Hughes suggested, and which I cancelled when we left the UK. No, things get done quickly here. You are taken seriously. Emily will be in safe hands. After the frustrations in England, finally I feel we might have a chance of an early diagnosis, and access to the all-important therapies.

By now, Emily is crawling around the room, becoming

fractious. It's time to leave. Anita is late for work, and I have the childminder waiting. We say our goodbyes to Dr Maier, who informs us we'll need to bring Emily back for some observation tests, and that she will email with details of the psychologist's appointment soon.

We speed out of there in the Polo, and in the rear-view mirror I catch my wife fighting back tears.

A long silence prevails until Anita, her eyes fixed on the road ahead, says: '"Retarded" is the correct word in German, it has none of the bad meaning it has in English.'

So she was translating for my benefit. It's all she says on the journey.

I'm dropped off by the *Bäckeri*, and haul Emily out of her seat into the buggy. Anita beeps the horn as she drives away, and I catch a glimpse of her big slate-grey eyes; a hopeful smile, and this reassures me. But after I've handed our daughter to the *Tagesmutter*, and I'm taking the toppling, decrepit wooden stairs two by two – fast, headlong – it's as if something heavy dislodges in my chest, and I fear I may start crying, and never stop.

Later that day, early evening. We are in the lounge, Anita back from work, both of us sitting on the sofa. Emily is still up, past her bedtime, stumbling around, spittle on her chin.

'So it's autism, then,' I say.

I glance at Anita, and her expression terrifies me. She's staring into space, weeping. She looks like someone sitting among the ruins of a destroyed building.

Emily surveys her mother curiously. I leave them in the lounge and walk slowly to the kitchen, close the door, and begin making dinner. I put on a CD, *Secrets of the Beehive* by David Sylvian and skip to the last track, 'Waterfront'. I know this will have the desired effect. The lines about memories, lost years, pouring rain. A dam bursts in my chest. I cry like I've never cried before in my life.

Then something cuts me short. That last, quiet, devastating couplet in which Sylvian questions whether 'our' love is strong enough.

I wipe my face with my sleeve. We need to be careful. People can, and do, break apart in situations like these.

14

Road

THE NEXT MORNING, I'm in a bad way. During breakfast I have to stop feeding Emily three times to choke back tears. She barely notices. On the kitchen table is a Polaroid photograph taken the day before by the neurologist. Emily's eyes are wide and beautiful, a sixties starlet.

Anita has already left for work, and I'm running late for Emily's first *ergothérapie* – occupational therapy – session. I half-clear the explosion of mess from the table, flannel Emily's face, brush her teeth, and after a struggle to put her into her snowsuit, mittens and boots, we're out on the freezing, icy street. I push the buggy fast, taking the road towards the centre of town.

A constant, questioning, hammering inner voice plagues me. What is her life going to be like? You can't wear a badge on a date, or a job interview that says, 'I'm autistic'. Will she ever *go* on a date, or have a job interview? What if she's nonverbal?

Of course, Emily may never speak.

Crossing a bridge over an *autobahn*, eight lanes of traffic rushing below, tears are spilling out again. I roar my guts out over the noise.

FUUUUUUUUUUUUUUUCCCKKKKKKKKKKKK

I'm quickly lost, looking for the address, cursing at cars and cyclists; yelling at the pelican crossings that allow vehicles to turn into your path when the green man is showing.

Will she ever call me 'Daddy'?

There are numerous junctions to negotiate. Big Mercedes and Audis park diagonally on the pavements, obstructing our path, their drivers popping into a *Bäkerei* for *Brötchen*.

Will she ever go to a normal school?

I stop a woman with jackdaw-black hair and ask for directions. She says I'm *almost* in the right place, I just need to turn left at the end, then right, then right again … She smiles indulgently at Emily. *Ah so*, I say, *vielen dank*.

Will she be teased and bullied at school?

The directions turn out to be wrong. Or I misunderstood them. We're nearly half an hour late, and the appointment is only 45 minutes in duration. Emily lost her mittens many streets back, and her hands are red and orange and swollen with the cold.

Will she ever build a snowman?

Finally, I find the road. Voltastraße, long and wide, with high tram-wires plunging into the distance. It's crammed with pedestrians, and I'm forced to slip into the bike lane. I gun the buggy hard into oncoming cyclists. *Move.*

Will she ever have any friends?

At last, I'm at the door, an expensive glass frontage. After three attempts at the buzzer, I heave the buggy in, then drag it up a short flight of stairs. My back and neck are soaked in sweat.

Will she need a helper in the supermarket?

The door to the clinic is open. I reverse the buggy in, apologise to the receptionist, who smiles, offers to make me coffee. The waiting room is clean and modern, mint green. IKEA pendant lights hang above the desk, on which sits a little jar of lollipops.

Will she be incontinent as an adult?

The young female therapist appears, and I introduce myself, apologising repeatedly for our lateness in pidgin German, while extracting a less-than-happy Emily from the buggy's straps. The woman smiles at Emily, says *Hallo*, remarks on her beauty. My daughter doesn't acknowledge her, but instead immediately stumbles off into one of the treatment rooms, startling a middle-aged patient. I catch her just before she pulls over a table of instruments.

Will she ever live an independent life?

The therapist says they prefer to conduct the sessions without the parents. That's fine, I say. I take a brief look at where Emily will spend 45 minutes every Wednesday morning. The room is littered with toys, a trampoline with a long blue ramp leading to it, a small hammock. As the door is closed, I glimpse my daughter, climbing slowly up the ramp, and a memory of a film returns, a beautiful, silent alien returning to the mother ship.

The next day, the despair has subsided somewhat. It felt like grief. But what species of grief was it? I recoil from the word – no one died. Emily is very much alive. To call it grief is an insult to parents who have had to bury a child. It is merely 'grief' for the child I'll never bring up. Either that, or self-pity. And this is something I've been wrestling with for the past year. Why us? I find myself thinking. And yet – why *not* us? Anita and I were unlucky, that's all. Someone's got to be. It is pure self-pity, that most shameful thing. Yet, self-pity is a valid human response, a genuine emotion in the aftermath of a tragedy. 'The question of self-pity' – almost the first words American essayist Joan Didion wrote after her husband died suddenly of a heart attack.

But this is surely a distraction from the main questions: how did we get to where we are now? Why was autism never mentioned by any medical professional in the UK? How has it taken a random search on the Internet one day to bring all of Emily's symptoms into sharp focus? Autism had been hiding there in plain sight, as the cliché has it, all along. Foolishly, I thought we'd got away with it; thought she was going to catch up, 'get better'. I assumed it was *all going to be OK*. I feel ill when I remember cancelling the MRI back in England. We could be six months ahead with the therapies Emily so desperately needs.

And now, each day, an apprehension dawns that this is only the start, that the first two years of her life, during which her symptoms could seem merely to be the sweet behaviour of a toddler – babbling, stumbling, dribbling – these may be the best years. What is to come may be ugly, and completely soul-destroying.

*

The one constant during this period are the songs I play for Emily on guitar. We're always in the living room, her wandering around among her scattered toys. First, I run the plectrum over the strings on the headstock, just above the nut. It makes a tinkly, musical box-like sound that always stops her in her tracks. Then a slow smile emerges. Is this a type of communication? I wonder. I'm trying to get through to her, to reach her. She still doesn't respond when I call her name. I'm not sure she knows she *has* a name, or what one is. I feel helpless when I repeat the word, over and over – 15, 20 times – and she doesn't react.

I start, as usual, with Pink Floyd's 'Wish You Were Here'. She walks around happily, smiling as the different sections of the song unfold. Once again, I note she seems to engage with music more than people. Why?

I'm suddenly aware of the obvious irony in the song's title. She doesn't seem to be properly 'here', present, much of the time. How I wish she was. But I also notice that she may have been bashing an object disconsolately, or stumbling from toy to toy, but when I start playing her concentration seems to improve. If she's showing frustration with an object, it all but disappears. And, studying her, I realise she is aware of me. She *is* 'here' – while the music plays, at least. Periodically, I will catch a small, sideways checking glance from her in my direction, accompanied by a sly smile, which I encourage. 'Do you like this one, Bear?' I ask. 'Here comes our verse – the one about the lost souls in the fishbowl!' It's as if the song is an invisible thread between us. A lifeline.

I decide to research genetics, a subject I know very little about. First, I Google 'genome', a word I think I vaguely know the meaning of, and the word Dr Hughes used in the meeting back in June. The genome is our full set of genes. We have 19,000 to 20,000. It was once thought we had 100,000, but through research the numbers are being revised down each year. That's how rapidly the science is evolving.

I find I'm brave enough to dig deeper. Something Dr Hughes said in the meeting, then expanded upon in his report, has been troubling me: 'It's possible there is a microdeletion or duplication on a neurodevelopmental locus'.

I Google 'microdeletion'.

A page of links to articles on microdeletion syndrome appears. Most of the pieces suggest that the condition is hereditary, but one says it can be caused by 'perinatal oxygen distress'.

I search for some more personal posts. Eventually, one catches my attention: a little girl who screamed for the first two years of her life, suffered from colic reflux, and displayed most of Emily's Global Developmental Delay symptoms. A thread below reveals testimonies from scores of parents who say they have 'the same child'. Most struggled to gain diagnoses, or have incomplete ones, or don't have one at all. The syndrome is related to autism. Most of the children are nonverbal, in special schools. Many of the families say how 'loving' and 'smiley' and 'happy' their children are, but accept they will never be able to live independent lives. The pain and anguish in some of the posts is almost impossible to bear. My hands are shaking as I read. If this is what Emily has, I don't know how we will possibly cope.

A sharp November afternoon. I take a walk with Emily in the buggy to *das Feld*, a plateau of arable land close to our neighbourhood. The air is damp, with traces of smoke; dead leaves lie in large clumps. Plough-lines take the eye to the misted horizon. It is a quiet place, a zone for contemplation.

There is despair in my heart. The 'grief' is back. The dream of having a normal child and a happy family life is over. And yet we still don't know for certain what the matter is, what is 'abnormal' about Emily. After a year of invasive tests, and with more to come, there is no definitive answer in sight, besides the spectre of autism. It's crushing me. It seems unthinkable that, only a matter of days ago, I believed Emily was getting better.

My thumbs are pinched with cold, causing me to worry about Emily's exposed digits. I check them occasionally, and her face. Her cheeks are red and her eyes are watering, spittle has dried on her chin. I feed her a piece of pretzel. She's taking in her surroundings, silently, as ever. Sealed in her – what? The only word I can think of is aloneness. Far away, on a path, a white dog – a Husky – is backlit by the low sun. It appears to be on fire. I point it out to her, but she doesn't follow my finger, of course.

I wonder if she will she remember any of this. Does she have 'a sense of a self that moves through time'? This is a phrase from a book I've been reading, Charles Fernyhough's *The Baby in the Mirror*, a developmental biography of his daughter's first three years. According to research, the first traceable memories occur at two and a half, when a child becomes 'properly verbal'. So if she has no language, will she have no memories? Another book on the bedside table is Oliver Sacks's *The Man Who Mistook His Wife for a Hat*, in which he quotes Luis Buñuel: 'Life without memory is no life at all ... Our memory is our coherence. Without it we are nothing'.

Our breath *shrrs* out in clouds.

I sense Emily beginning to tire of the buggy's confinement, so we head for home.

*

The only music I can listen to at the moment is wordless. Or rather, music where I can't make out the words. If that sounds eccentric, let me try to explain: Emily can't understand language, so why should I? The logic is twisted – there may *be* no logic – but nevertheless, this is the position I find myself in, as she approaches 25 months with no 'functional speech', in the jargon of developmental psychology. Perhaps the impulse is towards solidarity with her condition, to better comprehend how she experiences the world. Whatever the reason, I find that, lately, I seek out (wrong phrase – am *prone* to) music that works on an emotional level, that uses sound or silence, not words, to communicate; and which has a certain intensity. That, for me, can only mean one band: Talk Talk. (And yes, I'm aware of the irony of their name.)

I've been playing 1988's *Spirit of Eden* obsessively, the second album of the trilogy that began with *The Colour of Spring*. *Eden* has been a constant, generous companion for almost 30 years, its deep familiarity a source of comfort during difficult times.

A dramatic transformation in their sound has taken place since *The Colour of Spring*. The impressionistic template of 'April 5th' has been adapted to create a suite of unorthodox, mostly improvised 'songs', fusing jazz, classical, rock, and elements of ambient music. The first track, 'The Rainbow', begins with a funereal, unerring drum tattoo, played on a floor tom, reminiscent of the Velvet Underground. At specific points, this gives way to a startling change in tempo, accompanied by a key shift, a slippage unlike any that I can recall in music. It always puts me in mind of the moment a Super-8 film becomes stuck in the gate of a projector, a hole is burned, and rainbow colours spill out. Above this, singer Mark Hollis intones his largely indecipherable lyrics. Critics often say he mumbles or 'swallows' the words, and it's true – much of the time it's difficult to parse his meaning. The lyric sheet isn't helpful, either, written in his spidery, virtually illegible, backward-sloping hand. But one line is clear, the first line, which has a terrible resonance for me now. He distinctly says that his world has turned upside down. This is the world I'm living in at the moment, and 'The Rainbow' is both confirmation of – and insulation from – this place.

Recording for *Spirit of Eden* began in 1987, at Wessex Sound Studios, a converted church hall in leafy Highbury, north London. The band took nine months to complete the album. Stories about the sessions are legion, and have passed into post-rock lore. According to producer Phill Brown, there were no discussions as to musical direction beforehand, and very little was said each day in the studio. Wessex's cavernous main room was kept in near complete darkness – candles burning, incense lit – to create a disorientating, immersive atmosphere. Bassist Danny Thompson, who played on much of Nick Drake's work, was led to his amp in the gloom as if blindfolded. Mark Feltham, the harmonica player, was said to have been told not to venture outside of a chalk cross scrawled on the floor as he recorded his parts. One day, in a break caused by a heavy summer thunderstorm, Hollis suggested installing an oil-wheel

projector to create colourful psychedelic patterns on the walls
… And so the alchemical process continued, on EMI's generous
budget – *The Colour of Spring* had been a financial success –
often spending days recording a string section, only to keep
a mistake the cellist made, and wiping the rest. (It's estimated
that 80 per cent of what was put down onto tape was erased.)

What was Hollis searching for?

It's hard to tell, but the result was six uncategorisable pieces,
41 minutes of music, that combined passages of near silence
with sudden explosions of noise. For me, it is the silences that
are most interesting, where the 'personality' of Wessex's huge
main room, the old church hall, can be detected. All recording
engineers are aware of how the character of a particular room
can affect the character of the music. Wessex's studio one
conferred a unique sound, palpable even in the reverberations
from the sound of a chair creaking as a musician shifted to
become more comfortable …

Many years ago, in the mid-nineties, I found myself standing
in this room. My band was mixing at Wessex, and one day I
looked into the main studio, knowing that some of the great
punk albums had been recorded there. I wasn't aware that, only
a few years earlier, *Spirit of Eden* had been created there, too.
I opened a door, descended a wooden staircase, and stood for
a few hushed moments on the parquet floor. For some reason,
memories of primary school assemblies returned; hymns,
the smell of Pledge polish, the ghosts of flared and bearded
teachers. A decade later, I returned to Wessex, walking around
the perimeter hoping to catch a glimpse of the room again from
the outside. It was then that I learned the studio had closed,

the building divided into luxury apartments. But the thought that I once stood in the room gives me some comfort now, or a foothold on sanity, as I play 'I Believe In You', or 'Wealth', or 'The Rainbow' over and over again, unable to understand the words, in a world turned upside down.

Gradually, without any forward planning, communication rituals between Emily and I have begun to develop. The first was the Coming Home routine. We arrive at our front door after a walk where she will be absent, 'in her own world' – to adapt the phrase so often used to describe autistic children – and I put the double brake on the buggy. *Look-where-we-are!* I sing, to a tune made up on the spot. *Look-where-we-are!* Emily becomes excited, and starts kicking her feet. I take out my keys; show them to her. *Key, key, key!* I sing, this time to the melody of 'Three Blind Mice', in the hope that she might copy the word. Then I operate the lock, push the door open, put the stopper down and heft the buggy with Emily's weight in it up the first short flight of steps.

She looks up at me expectantly, enjoying seeing me upside down. This is the first piece of communication. Then, when I've stationed the buggy beside the second flight of stairs, I retrace my steps, looking back theatrically over my shoulder every so often to ensure her gaze is upon me. I have her full attention now. Maximum eye contact, the most she will give in an entire day sometimes. She starts to giggle. I close the front door, lower myself with one deliberate, exaggerated movement, like a big cartoon cat or dog – and run as fast as I can towards her, arms flailing wildly above my head. She's laughing hysterically by now. I pounce on her, tickle her once, twice, three times. She squeals with delight. When she's calmed down, I unhook the buggy's straps and haul her out for the fireman's lift upstairs. As we ascend, she makes loud, high-pitched, word-like sounds, enjoying testing out the reverb in the stairwell. I'm not sure the neighbours do as much.

There are other rituals, too. Showing her the empty bowl after she's eaten her yoghurt. *Gone, gone, gone!* I sing. Her reaction: turning away to giggle, a Shirley Bassey shape. Or when I walk into her room brushing my teeth in the morning with the electric toothbrush. Her face lights up. If it gets a reaction, it's added to the setlist.

*

'Put your hands around her arms, like a belt,' says the doctor as the instrument goes in.

An audiology appointment for Emily in central Frankfurt: late November.

In seconds, her face is purple. She shrieks and cries in outrage. When the ordeal is over, I take her to the consulting room's narrow window to recover for a few minutes.

The ear examinations have been mercifully brief, but predictably unpleasant.

After making some notes in a folder, the doctor – possibly my age, firm handshake, perfect English – speaks. He suspects the central nerve in her ear may have been damaged through lack of oxygen at birth, and needs to do further tests. It's just an idea, he says. This could be the reason for her delayed speech.

We're here again.

I'm suddenly stricken with the fear that the phrase 'lack of oxygen at birth' always gives me in one of these rooms.

This muddies the waters, I say. We were hoping for a routine appointment to check on the fluid after the procedure, after which we'd exit with a prognosis that her hearing was improving.

He proposes an investigation under melatonin. This will induce a narcosis to keep her head still. I agree to it, but then take the opportunity to tell him as much background information about Emily as I can: the year of tests in England, the therapies – and the fact that autism has now been put forward by a neurologist here. He listens earnestly as I speak; doesn't dismiss the autism theory. I have the impression he's an ally, he wants to solve the mystery as much as I do.

'We must be patient,' he says as I'm leaving with Emily over my shoulder, 'gather all the facts first.'

Later, after I've dropped her at the childminder's, I go for a long, aimless walk. I need to get out; think. Heavy rain is coming down, soaking me in seconds. I've left the house without a coat.

So maybe the fluid wasn't the reason for Emily's lack of response to speech, but nerve damage. Or she has microdeletion syndrome. Or she's autistic. Or both. Who knows? We've gone off on yet another tangent.

I pause on the *autobahn* bridge, in the drenching storm, watching the vehicles roar and zip below – cars, trucks, tankers, all displacing immense amounts of rainwater as they hurtle towards Cologne or Amsterdam, and I wonder what it would be like to fall.

Fall into their path.

15

The Dark Is Rising

ONE WEEK LATER, we have a second meeting with the neurologist. The observation tests. We drive out to the children's hospital – Anita, Emily and I – crossing the boat-dotted river once again, past stands of alder and birch, their autumn colours muted now.

We park, and wait patiently in the cool, stylish, empty reception area. It feels more like an airport departure lounge than a hospital.

Dr Maier appears, as friendly as before, and welcomes us into her consulting room. She is still wearing matching purples, and still using the word 'retarded', or 'retardation', when referring to our daughter. She warns us, with a serious look, that 'this is not going to go away in the next year', and to find Emily a place at an *Integrativ* – integrated – kindergarten for special needs children as soon as possible.

So this is what she is now, officially, I think to myself. Special needs. I recall Anita spitting the word back in April. *Special*.

'Labelled already'. It's a mark of how far we've come that this phrase doesn't elicit a reaction from either of us.

We discuss a one-day battery of hospital tests, most of which Emily has already undergone in the UK. But I'm resigned to the fact that she will have to endure them all again, here in Germany. We tell the neurologist we're eager for our daughter to have the MRI, to finally uncover what the problem is.

Emily's mood is deteriorating, so the observation tests are carried out swiftly: eyes, reflexes, a rattle to assess her hearing, a tape measure around her head. She's stripped down to her nappy, and I feel sad and desperate, as I always do when this happens. Finally, when Emily's crying becomes too much, I take her outside and walk her up and down the long deserted corridors, leaving Anita to conclude the meeting. When we return, I notice a child's drawing of a lion on the wall besides Dr Maier's office, signed Isabella – Emily's middle name. *Emily Isabella, the Lionheart.*

After a few moments, Anita emerges from the room. We shake hands with Dr Maier, and make our way to the Polo. I sit in the back beside Emily, so I can hold her hand, and sing the songs that will calm her. 'Row Your Boat', 'The Wheels On The Bus', 'Old MacDonald', 'Ten Green Bottles'.

This is not going to go away in the next year.

I feel wretched.

For the first few moments in the car there is silence. Then Anita says, 'Well?'

'Well, what?' I say.

'There's a long journey ahead.'

'I don't like the word journey,' I say, 'it implies a destination.'

What am I talking about? What pompous nonsense.

I'm silent once more, stroking Emily's hand.

'When you were out of the room, Dr Maier said Em was a mystery.'

I can't think of a reply. The sky has fallen in.

'Don't write her off yet,' Anita says. '*Hope dies last.*'

We cross the low, misted River Main. Emily's tiny hand feels smooth, like a pebble found on the shore, yet it is light, lighter than air somehow, and warm. Weightless.

A schoolgirl on a bike – black coat, blonde hair – flies past on the other side of the road. Emily will never do this, I think, and my breath is ripped away. By a roundabout, I see a group of younger children standing with their teacher, their colourful rucksacks in a pile. The sight crushes me. Everywhere, futures are closing for her.

Anita breaks the silence, and a tense, surreal conversation ensues. Irreversible brain damage or autism? Or some other syndrome? A hierarchy of tragedy is emerging, I say. An array of hopeless outcomes.

'You've got to have faith,' says Anita.

Anger rises in me.

'I do have faith.'

I have faith in Emily – who she actually is, not a 'normal' version of her. But I don't say this, I just stroke her hand, and stare at the numberless trees in the dark forest – so evenly spaced – flashing by, flashing by.

The following weekend, we have friends over for lunch – Sophie, her partner Dennis, and their daughters, Lina, three, and Amelie, one. We sit in the lounge eating Anita's homemade soup with *Brötchen*. There is a cheerful atmosphere. Afterwards, in hats and coats and gloves, we go to the playground in the wood. Sullen winter light pierces the aspens. The freezing wind causes falling leaves to shoot about like birds. There is cold in my bones, and misery in my heart.

'It's like a proper family Saturday!' says Anita, smiling her broad, toothsome smile.

But I am locked in a cell of depression, virtually mute, avoiding all conversation. It's the comparison, especially with Amelie, who is half Emily's age, that I can't seem to overcome. I survey the scene: our children playing on the swings, the slide, in the sandpit. It *should* be like a proper family Saturday, a happy winter outing, but I can't feel it. I wish I could deal with the situation as Anita is doing, bravely and brightly, but all I can see are the trees losing leaves, the light draining from the afternoon, and Emily in her own world.

We move to the path that hugs the stream. One of Sophie's friends – another mum – out walking with her three-year-old daughter, Mila, joins us. The child appraises me with serious, vigilant eyes. Kids, I realise – normal kids – are like writers: they notice everything. I've been reading more about this. It's because they're learning from you, trying to read your mind. Autistic children are thought to have 'mind-blindness', no feeling for, or concept of other minds. I think back to the level, disconcerting stares of Emily's playmates that greeted me each morning at the nursery in Surbiton. They were looking for clues from a grown-up, any sign or tip that would assist them in understanding the confusing social world of adult human beings.

Meanwhile, Emily gazes off into the distance, or stumbles down a bank towards the stream like a drunkard. We call after her but she is oblivious. I give chase, and catch her just before she plunges into the water.

Eventually, we wander back to the apartment. I watch as the older girls, Lina and Mila, pair up to cross a road. They run ahead, then stop at the curb, waiting obediently for the parental command. I experience a tremor of fear. Emily, in that situation, wouldn't respond to any sort of direction at all. 'Compliance' it's called, in the jargon. The comprehension of words such as 'no', 'stop' and 'go'.

Worse is to come when we return.

The kids are given free rein to play in the lounge. The older ones adore the ball pond in the Wendy house, and soon it's pandemonium in there, a lottery tombola. I study Amelie, on her own in another part of the room, as she raises herself to a standing position, knees bent: the child's weightlifter move. She can do this already, at just one. She wanders over to Emily and shoves her gently, imploring her to react. Emily becomes upset, so I intervene. I pick up the small, red charity shop tambourine and start playing a confident, even, 4/4 rhythm. A Tamla Motown beat. The other children's faces pop out of the Wendy house and stare up at me in awe, their avid, expectant eyes locked onto mine. Suddenly, I'm a wizard, a Pied Piper.

Emily stumbles off, but then returns, and plays happily alongside Amelie for a while. I crouch down in order to demonstrate a toy: a moulded plastic giraffe. It comes with small cubes that need to be placed in a trapdoor in the animal's head, until there are too many, and they are disgorged through the feet with a little flurry of musical notes. I watch, gloatingly almost, as I know Amelie will quickly deduce what to do. She picks up the cubes and places them in the opening until they tumble down the giraffe's neck, and spill out of the hatch below. *Tra-la-la!* She does it again, then again, with a sort of pedantic, pragmatic absorption, a mathematician solving an easy problem. Emily has never been able to do this, not even close. It's one of the occupational therapy exercises, putting a small object into a larger one, a hoop into a bowl, say.

What is wrong with her brain that she cannot comprehend this? *Why* can't she do this simple task? Why?

I sit down on the sofa next to Dennis. I'm afraid the other parents know there is something wrong – we haven't said anything about the hospital appointments with the neurologist, the upcoming tests with the developmental psychologist, but they must have noticed Emily's difference. I watch them furtively, in my peripheral vision, alert to any sign that they suspect.

I watch the other children, too, absorbed in their play, Emily excluded, wandering around listlessly, clutching the tambourine. Waves of panic keep rising in me.

She's autistic, I'm certain of it.

The waves keep coming.

She's autistic.

This is torture.

Amelie starts playing with a newspaper. The broadsheet, *Die Zeit*. Dennis, her amiable, slightly built dad, who has his short legs stretched out on the sofa next to me, looks up from his iPhone.

'She's going to be an intellectual!' he says, grinning, and goes back to his screen.

The remark wounds me. It's not his fault. Then Amelie raises herself to the First Steps Baby Walker and starts to push it across the lounge. Dennis looks up from his phone again, and says, nonchalantly, like someone noticing a shop they hadn't seen before on the High Street, 'Oh, that's new. She couldn't do that before.'

How casually they take normal development for granted, I think, bitterly.

And every time one of the children points at something it's like being run through by the blade of a knife.

Just at that moment, I hear Sophie, who hasn't seen Emily for a few months, say, 'Gosh, Em is just so *pretty*! Like from a fairy tale or film.'

So it is the prettiest one who is the condemned one, is it? My Prettiest Star, my golden daughter. What a cruel trick, God. What a cruel God you are. Do you remember my prayer, the one I said a lifetime ago, back in Surbiton, after the pregnancy test, kneeling on the hard wooden floor of the lounge, in front of St Mark's church spire? *Please, don't let the kid have anything wrong with it.*

Well I say to you now in my heart: *Fuck you, God.*

Fuck you.

The next day, at breakfast, I'm in a black, morbid depression. I'm aware that this is not useful in any way, but I'm powerless to control it. So what do we do now? I ask Anita, who is calmly feeding Emily. Wait for whatever life sentence is in store for her, and us? Who are we now? Parents, or carers? I feel as if a new description of ourselves is starting to emerge, a new identity: the parents – and carers – of an intellectually disabled daughter.

In a perverse way there is a sort of relief. I'm set free from a grand illusion, the myth of the perfect child. This is what the last two ghastly weeks have been about – a massive recalibration of the future.

I hear my pulse loud in my ears when I think about the future. The question keeps reasserting itself: who will look after Emily when we're gone? Who will protect her? But we can't be sure the future holds terrible things for her, I have to tell myself, no one can. It's here I realise my coping mechanism is bizarre. My way of dealing with a potentially catastrophic situation is to fear the worst, then, if it doesn't happen there is a reprieve. Strangely, I find I can handle despair, but not hope.

One afternoon, not long after the terrible family Saturday, I come across a photocopy of Emily's labour and delivery summary from the hospital birth notes. I skim-read it, looking at the boxes that have been ticked.

Presentation and position at delivery; mode of delivery; Apgar score: 7 (1 min), 7 (5 min), 9 (10 mins). Resuscitation: yes.

Resuscitation?

There is a slightly scratchy tick in the bottom right-hand corner of the box. This was never mentioned.

I read on. *Method: IPPV.*

What is IPPV?

I decide to Google it, with all the knotted-stomach dread that accompanies such investigations.

It stands for Intermittent Positive Pressure Ventilation, often used when there has been a meconium, or after a forceps birth. Emily had both … Another page is titled 'neo-natal resuscitation errors'. I take a long breath, and click. A page from an American law firm's site comes up. It's harrowing, white-knuckle reading. 'Intubation' seems to be the most risky procedure: the swift insertion of an endotracheal tube into the mouth and then into the airway to assist breathing. A 20-second window that could either destroy the child's brain – wipe the hard drive – or save its life. Christ. No one would ever have children if they read this sort of stuff first. That's why I never did.

I look back at the birth notes. 'Intubation' is un-ticked, but then other parts of the page are incomplete, too. So Emily was resuscitated. I did not know this. I know her crying was late, and weak. I remember that. But not much else – I was borne up on a wave of euphoria, elated that she was alive after the ordeal of the labour.

I put the photocopy down. This could be an important discovery.

Or it could be nothing.

The day of Emily's hospital tests arrives. A 24-hour overnight stay: the EEG, an ultrasound, and the MRI brain scan, the procedure that we opposed so vehemently, then acquiesced to, is to take place tonight. Tomorrow we will discover if her brain is damaged.

I rise at 5:30am and feed Emily porridge with mashed banana. She is happy and co-operative, if slightly confused by this night-time treat. As I load the spoon, she acknowledges me from time to time with beaming grins, and I take her through what's going to happen. I'm pretty sure she doesn't understand, but I do it anyway.

Her little feet in grippy socks are resting on my knees. Suddenly, I feel an overwhelming tenderness for her; an intense ache in my chest that lasts for a few unbearable seconds. I hope nothing goes wrong. Physiotherapist Jane's words about the general anaesthetic return: *you don't want her to be the one-in-whatever-it-is that has an adverse reaction*, but I try to put them out of my mind.

There's only accommodation for one parent at the hospital, so it's been agreed I stay at home. I help Anita carry Emily, the buggy and their numerous bags down the stairs. Outside, the temperature is minus eight. There are icicles forming on the boot of the car. The doors have a slippery carapace of ice, which creak, then snap open. A high-flying bird overhead in the chill, inky sky startles Emily, and she looks up, her eyes wide. I hug them both.

'Think of us,' Anita says.

And then they are gone.

16

Watching You
Without Me

THE NEXT MORNING, I'm woken by a text from Anita. The MRI went smoothly. There were no complications from the anaesthetic. Relief floods through me. But could I come up to the hospital now? The scan took place at 2am, and they're exhausted.

Half an hour later I'm on a train, crossing the river. I'm elated at the news, and thinking excitedly of my wife and child, eager to see them.

As the train pulls further away from the suburbs, sunlight flashes between apartment buildings. A harsh frost shows on passing fields. The carriage becomes emptier and emptier. Bike shops, fitness studios, funeral parlours start to appear. Small-town Germany.

I alight at the correct stop, find the *Kinderkrankenhaus*, and take a lift to the sixth floor. *Station sechs*. I push through a white double door into a light-filled room. Emily, wearing a little gown, is standing in a cot. She looks tired, but her face cracks into a smile when she sees me. A reckless feeling of joy holds me in its grip. My emotions feel amplified; too close to the surface. I notice she has traces of glue in her hair from the EEG electrodes. Anita embarks on a resume of the night's events, but I'm distracted. Outside, in the corridor, disabled children in wheelchairs are passing by.

'Honestly, I've seen some things here,' Anita says. 'Be thankful for what you've got.'

'Well, no one's here because their kid is OK,' I reply.

Why can't I stop? Why must I always steer towards an argument?

I move over to the cot and try to soothe Emily to sleep. Anita goes to the doorway to check her phone. Just at that moment, a young man with a trim beard and a grey-and-white-striped sweatshirt stops to talk to her. Although dressed casually, he has the air of someone important ... the consultant paediatrician perhaps? There is a brief exchange. Yes, yes it is the consultant paediatrician. I can't hear what they're saying, and, anyway, it's in German. Could these be the results? Abruptly, the doctor walks away, and Anita steps back into the room smiling, her eyes bursting with good news.

It is indeed the results, and they are startling.

Emily's MRI is completely normal. 'Clear', in the doctor's words. So there was no brain damage caused by lack of oxygen during the labour, the birth or resuscitation. I'm dazed by this information, but also enormously relieved.

I lift Emily out of the cot; stand her up on the floor, crouch down next to her, hug her.

The news, although marvellous, somehow confuses matters even further.

'So what *is* going on in that noodle of yours?' I ask, my mouth touching her hair. I kiss her warm forehead. I can smell almonds or biscuits. Her Emily smell. 'What *is* going on in there?'

*

December. It's darker now at 8am, on the childminder run. The depression is back: a dreadful, dark well or vortex that I can't seem to climb out of. I have the urge to train, go running, shave my head – all displacement activities that I know are associated with controlling the uncontrollable. I'm foul to live with. I'm drinking too much wine in the evening. Anita says I seem so angry all the time. We've been arguing more and more – it's madness, when Emily's wellbeing is our common goal. She says I need therapy, counselling, for what we're going through. Perhaps I do.

I point the buggy down the vertiginous cut by the church, and run. Emily yowls with joy. The last yellow leaf-fall is underfoot. *December will be magic again.*

Will it? Christmas soon. Merry Christmas. I can't see anything merry about it.

So the MRI scan was clear. I know I should be pleased about this, but I can't be, somehow. Nothing has changed. What developmental disorder *does* our daughter have, then? On a mundane, practical level, we need some sort of diagnosis to be eligible for an *Integrativ* kindergarten.

Some days it feels as if this is all too much to bear.

I yell at a driver approaching a junction too quickly. I curse at cars that don't stop at the zebra crossings for us.

And this place: our neighbourhood. Germany. I'm questioning why have we come here. Yes, it is probably the best place for Emily, from a medical point of view, but for the first time I feel homesick. I read something online about the Kingsland Road, and felt a sharp pang, a longing for London. I find myself wondering how long we will have to live here.

What's more, I can't find work. I've placed advertisements, joined Facebook groups, everything I can think of. I must have been into all the bars in Frankfurt asking for a gig. Nothing doing. And if they do hire bands they tell me they pay in 'beer and pizza'. There is something else, too. I've discovered there was a thriving live scene here until, a few years ago, the copyright laws changed. A separate licence for each song is now needed to perform it in public. This explains the proliferation of tribute bands: they only need 15 to 20 licences and they're set up in business. If only I'd researched this properly before the move, but we left so abruptly there wasn't time.

So far, I've played two gigs with one of Anita's work colleagues. A local pub that brazenly host 'open-mic' nights using professional musicians as a way of gaining a night's entertainment for free. A hat went round. We ended up with 30 euros between us.

The outcome is that, for now, for the first time in my life, I am living off a partner's means.

*

Everywhere I look I see fathers and daughters. In the newsagent, a poster shows a middle-aged dad with his teenage daughter looking at something on a laptop. Someone on Twitter has posted a tweet that reads 'Happy twenty-first', accompanied by two photographs. One is of a little girl climbing a tree, maybe seven years old; the other is of a beautiful young woman in a blue dress, smiling, leaning in to kiss a proud-looking man in his forties, clearly her dad. It feels like an axe to my heart. Emily's future seems to have been cancelled.

Any reference to girls older than Emily hurts. Accounts of daughters drawing, painting, baking, playing with pipe-cleaners, finding costumes in dressing-up baskets, needing lifts to concert rehearsals maul me ... One dad, in an article about his eight-year-old, writes about her singing a song from a film: *I'm off on a remarkable adventure!* 'All eight-year-olds are,' he says. All? I have that awful feeling again: Emily may never do this. It feels as if she is being robbed of her entire childhood.

One day I come across an article in some online magazine. The mother's tone, when referring to her three-year-old daughter, I find insufferably smug. The little girl can name all her dolls, speak in good sentences, insists on wearing a red tutu when dancing to her favourite song ... Suddenly, I feel the urge to smash my laptop to pieces. I hurl it from the desk in a fit of pure envy.

And yet, and yet ...

Playing with Emily today, landing Alby, the soft-toy albatross I bought in a Surbiton charity shop one day on the roof of the Wendy house. Her squeals of surprise, delight. Or feeding her at teatime, her feet on my knees, smiling with her mouth full. Or her practising high-pitched notes at top volume, 'singing', expressing how happy she feels.

She *is* happy.

If Emily can be happy, then surely I have a duty to be, too.

We get through a weekend at Anita's parents. Playing with Emily's young cousins in the lounge is the hardest part. The bizarre thought occurs that these children – these *talking* children – are people, and Emily is … something else. But what? An alien? I remember one recent sleepless night of terrible thoughts, coming to terms with all that was happening, and in the morning feeling distant, disconnected from Emily, as if she'd changed, or been someone else all along. A stranger. It felt as if I'd somehow made a mistake in my evaluation of her, and couldn't enjoy being her father anymore. Yet when I went to her room the next morning to wake her, there she was, standing up in her cot in the sleeping bag, smiling expectantly. The same old Emily, happy and affectionate; a personality. A person.

Driving back on the Sunday, I ask Anita how she would feel if Emily could never say a word, for the whole of the rest of her life. As the question leaves my mouth, my heart flutters in my chest. To hear my secret fear vocalised is shocking. Something similar happened last week, speaking to my brother on the phone. I said, 'We may have to accept Emily is …' and, softly, he finished the sentence: 'Mentally disabled.' I froze in horror to hear thoughts so often struggled with in private out in the open, on someone else's lips. It made them seem all the more real.

Andrew, Carrie and Billy come to visit. It's the first time I've seen Andrew since the holiday in Gran Canaria. We have a *Pilsner*, or two, to celebrate, then, with our families, head to the Christmas market in Frankfurt. I'm anxious because of the recent attack on one in Berlin. Ironically, after the worry about terrorism in London, Isis seem to have switched their operation to central Europe.

Carols and folk songs play, the chilly air reeks of burnt almonds, cooking pork and *Glühwein*. The kids ride on a carousel. Anita holds Emily, who spins around with wide, puzzled eyes. Billy, who is two-and-a-half now, has three turns at the wheel of a fire engine, his expression eager, serious.

In the evening, after a feast of Greek food and much wine, the video of Emily's first birthday is played. Lights are dimmed, and the film is projected onto one of the apartment's huge white walls. The ghostly images play in the dark. There is Emily in the villa, smaller, hair lighter, in a high chair. There is Billy sitting next to her. Andrew asks him questions. *Where's your tum-tum?* After some thought, Billy pats his belly. *Where's your bum-bum?* He pats his behind. Emily looks on, hands flapping, crying.

Some more of Emily's test results have arrived. I've asked Dr Maier to call me at home on the landline. I'm nervous, and my hands tremble slightly as I pick up the ringing telephone. She sounds open and friendly, yet professional – as she is in person – and there is a smile in her voice. Perhaps the news won't be bad. After a few pleasantries, she begins a summary of the findings.

'There was one result from the genetic test, but we need to wait for the rest.'

'OK,' I say, making a mental note to return to this. First, I want to confirm the main event. 'And the consultant told us the MRI was normal?'

'Yes, all clear. No damage due to lack of oxygen or bleeding. We can also see if the brain is not as big as others, or if something is missing, etc.'

Hold on. Something is troubling me. They did do an fMRI – a functional MRI – didn't they?

'Oh, no!' Dr Maier sounds alarmed, scandalised even. 'We only do that before a surgery or something.'

Carefully, I explain how there is new science that shows the fMRI can detect autism with 97 per cent accuracy. But she is adamant that, currently, the only diagnosis for the condition possible is from a behavioural or clinical test. Typical of doctors, I want to say, following the rules, until she asks: 'Where did you read this?'

I think back. It was part of a Google search that dredged up an article from ... the *Daily Mail*. I now recall the tone, another 'medical miracle' piece. And the fMRIs, if I remember correctly, had all been paid for privately in the United States, probably by parents as desperate as we are.

I burn with shame at my own gullibility.

'There is no direct connection between MRI and autism,' she asserts, recovering her composure. 'We see that Emily has a behavioural *retardation* similar to autism, that's all.'

That word again. I'll never get used to it.

I try another tack.

'So we can't do anything, then,' I say, 'in terms of actual action – therapies – we just have to wait and see if it is autism?'

And I can't believe I've used this phrase, after all I've read online about not accepting a 'wait-and-see diagnosis'.

'No,' Dr Maier replies, 'we can still pursue therapies, but a clinical psychologist will have to assess Emily first, after which she can be referred to the autism centre in Frankfurt.'

For a moment, I feel reassured. Then she returns to the test results. The bloods, thyroid, ultrasound, were all 'totally normal'. The EEG, too, 'important, if they don't speak,' she adds.

'You said there was one genetic result?' I ask.

'Yes, Fragile X syndrome, seldom seen with a female. We have lots of children here with it. It's linked to autism.'

'OK ...'

My skin prickles.

'She doesn't have that. But we're still waiting for the main genetic test, the CGH micro-array analysis, which may point to other syndromes.'

I can sense the call concluding, so I make one last attempt to see if she will be drawn out. Does she have any specific idea as to what is actually wrong with Emily?

'No specific ideas, no. Apart from the autism hunch. We have to wait until we've gathered all the information, then go from there. I'm curious to see the pathologic results from the CGH. I don't want there to be anything found, of course ... Sometimes we don't find the answer. In many cases there is no reason.'

The conversation ends with me thanking her for her time, and wishing her a happy Christmas.

'And to you. Say hello to your wife,' she says.

I put the phone back in the cradle. One year on from the first paediatrician appointment in England, and it feels as if we're still no nearer to an answer.

*

The winter solstice. After I've dropped Emily at the childminder's I make my way to the bridge over the *autobahn*. I've been coming here more and more often in the past weeks, to experience the curious feeling the place gives me. The contrary motion of walking above eight lanes of roaring traffic, at a 90-degree angle, induces a sort of vertigo, and a fight-or-flight response. One tenses as if in proximity to a dangerous natural feature, a flooding river or weir. Down below, red points of light flow away from me, yellow towards me. The noise is huge. I stop, stand by the railings, and peer over the brink.

When I return, I check my inbox. There's a communication from Dr Maier. The body of the email begins in the subject bar, and is truncated: 'Dear Mr Cook, I just received one other result from the Ge …'

I know that 'Ge' has to be short for 'Genetics'. With an elevated heart rate, I click on the mail.

There was something 'conspicuous' found on one of Emily's genetic test results. I'm pretty sure that 'conspicuous' is a medical euphemism for abnormal. She wants Anita and I to give a blood sample, to check if either of us have the same feature.

A few days later we are sitting in the local GP's clean, spacious office. It looks more like a room in a bank or an insurance company. There is a broad, steel-and-glass desk with a black blotter. A selection of expensive-looking fountain pens. The space seems too un-medical for blood to be taken, but that is what we're here for. Only a mechanical bed in a corner covered by a paper sheet says it's a surgery. We are in two chairs facing the desk, waiting for the *Ärtzin* – the female doctor – to appear, an odd German custom, it seems. The receptionist calls you, then you wait again in an empty room. We could steal all her pens.

She arrives, a tall woman wearing a stiff, calf-length white coat. Rimless spectacles, dark bob with traces of grey, alarmingly large, scrubbed hands. She asks a few preliminary questions in German, then indicates that I'm first. I hop up onto the bed. She's good. Quick. I have a sudden flashback to pushing Emily in the buggy through Surbiton, showing her off. *Look at what my genes have produced.* Then it's Anita's turn. We're both nervous, and end up sitting in each other's chairs.

The wine-dark blood lies in two clear tubes capped with blue stoppers. The doctor writes on them neatly with a fountain pen, and puts them into larger white plastic bottles. Do they contain genetic secrets we'd rather were not revealed? Do they contain the key to Emily's condition?

*

'Look at the birds … look at the *sky*!'

Her voice is small but surprisingly assured.

I have another dream in which Emily can talk. We're in the bedroom of my childhood home in Hitchin, by the window. She is standing with her eyes closed, when she suddenly opens them and speaks.

The scene jump-cuts, and we're on an old, heavy iron-framed bicycle, touring around the town, her little hands on my back. She tells me about her thoughts and feelings during the past year, all we have missed.

'There's so much to catch up on!' I say.

The following morning, at breakfast, I tell Anita about the

dream. She says it was 'cute'. I can tell she believes Emily will talk, eventually.

I feel exasperation rising.

'I thought the dream was terrible, actually,' I say, 'because there's a good chance she will never speak. Is she just going to pull it out of the bag when she's four?'

Silence.

We argue horribly later. Somehow, in the tragedy that seems to be engulfing us, we've lost any sort of perspective or control. Sometimes, I have the terrifying feeling that Anita doesn't want to be with me anymore, that she no longer loves me.

Four days later. Anita is bouncing a delighted Emily on the bed. I crawl around to the other side and leap up like a mad dog. Emily explodes with laughter. I grab her ankles and pull her incrementally towards me. *Gotcha!* It's infectious, we're all laughing now, overborne with joy. Anita takes hold of Emily's hands and bounces her higher and higher, our daughter cackling and screaming, her wild blonde hair leaping about. Then I grab her and throw her onto the bed, which she finds hysterically funny. She makes a mad-dash crawl for the edge. I catch her just before she falls to the floor. *Oh no, oh no!*

Then the bouncing starts all over again.

How being a parent completes me. How I wished for it at 40, single, losing hope; looking down into a Surbiton courtyard at a couple spinning their daughter around and around. And now I am a parent. But it is not as I imagined it would be.

17

Carolyn's Fingers

MAYBE I DON'T need therapy, just that 'good medicine': music. I've barely listened to any since the autumn, apart from Nick Drake and Talk Talk. It's January, the month in which I always play Cocteau Twins; one album in particular – *Treasure*, the LP I had on my headphones as I rested on my midnight walk home in Church Passage, Surbiton.

The record always reminds me uncomfortably of the teenage crush I had on the singer, Elizabeth Fraser (I even wrote a terrible song for her, 'Elizabeth', aged 16). I was obsessed with her voice – an unclassifiable, apparently self-taught soprano – a sound capable of expressing a formidable range of emotions. In it one could hear suffering, joy, anger, pious romantic longing – but never understand a single word, as she sang in an invented language. (Well, some words and phrases were comprehensible, 'follow the arrow', 'listen to me', 'sugar hiccup after Cheerios' – at least that's what I thought she was singing.) Of course, this only added to her mysterious allure.

It's her voice I need at the moment, like Hollis's, another 'wordless' means of communication. From an interview, I learn that Fraser suffered from stage fright, and lacked the courage to sing in English; thought it would be too revealing. Instead, she invented Latinate terms, took snippets of foreign languages from dictionaries or cookery books. Pieced together at random, they formed a glossolalia that, she insisted, had no meaning at all until sung. (This led to many amusing translations on foreign lyric sheets, and, more than once, to me playing the vinyl at the wrong speed in my adolescent bedroom, not noticing anything was wrong.)

Watching Fraser sing live – as I was lucky enough to do only once, at Kilburn National Ballroom, 1986 – her eyes wide, jaw lowered, shoulders trembling, was an unforgettable experience. Several times she punched herself in the throat to produce effects from the larynx (and each time, with an eye on our future together, I said to myself: *No Liz, please don't do that*). But it was the emotion in her voice that connected. She wasn't a singer who interacted with the audience or smiled as she sang, 'feeling the words'. She didn't need to. You understood with your gut.

Cocteau Twins were not twins at all but a couple from Grangemouth, Stirlingshire, a small town on the east coast of Scotland. (Fraser's partner was guitarist and producer Robin Guthrie.) Many people, myself included, were surprised to find that they swore like dockers in their interviews with the music press, something at variance with their high-art 4AD record sleeves, and Guthrie's dense, ambient sound design, which invariably elicited adjectives such as 'shimmering', 'ethereal', or 'God-like' from journalists. An early standout example of their unique style is a track they recorded under the name This Mortal Coil, a cover of Tim Buckley's 'Song To The Siren'. The piece has deep emotional meaning for me, and would be too powerful at the moment. I'm building up to it. For now, the chilly, amniotic currents of *Treasure* will have to do.

One afternoon, not long after New Year, I pick Emily up from the childminder and we go for a short walk. I don't feel like returning to the apartment immediately. We roam the streets, until, on a broad *Allee*, I notice a middle-aged woman wearing a bright red scarf and matching spectacle frames. She is powerless to stop herself smiling, and appears to have something extremely important to tell us. I wonder if I know her, but I'm certain I've never seen her before. When she reaches the buggy, she stops, looks down at Emily and utters a phrase in German. I hear the word '*Puppe*' – doll. When she guesses that I'm English, she says: 'Ah! She's just like a lovely little doll! So beautiful!'

So that's all it was, she just wanted to dote.

'A little doll!' she repeats, as she straightens her scarf and, still smiling, prepares to leave us. I suppress the desperate thoughts – that my daughter can't reply, probably doesn't even know what a doll is – and smile a weak 'thank you' back.

The meeting with the developmental psychologist at the children's hospital arrives. Dr Schroeder is young and friendly, with kind, pale blue eyes, and a voluminous tasselled cotton scarf wrapped around her neck in the German fashion. She agrees to speak English where possible for the duration of the meeting. Emily, in her best pink party dress, sits with Anita on a playmat in the centre of the room. I take a seat opposite the psychologist's desk.

The questions first, always the questions. Does Emily have any words yet? Does she point, draw your attention to something? What sounds does she make? What is her eye contact like? How does she react to other children? Does she have any fears? Finally, she asks, *what do you like most about her?* It's a disarming enquiry. I have to concentrate to keep my voice steady.

'Early on,' I say, 'it was clear she had a sense of humour; she smiled and laughed a lot, which seemed to me such a sophisticated response to life … Aristotle once said …' I quickly glance at Dr Schroeder to gauge her reaction. She's looking at me intently. 'Aristotle once said that the moment a child first laughs is when its soul is formed.'

I trail off; try to compose myself, then continue: 'She never lost it, her laugh, I mean, so I guess if I had to say the thing I like the *most* about her is her wonderful sense of humour, of fun. Her personality. Her spirit.'

I can feel tears hot and close behind my eyes.

'Her soul.'

Dr Schroeder makes some notes with a blue fountain pen, and tentatively introduces the subject of autism. Within minutes, she is talking frankly about the condition. Emily will have many behavioural tests to complete.

I notice Anita, playing with Emily, her face reddening, tears coming.

I ask about language.

'In your experience, if it is autism, will speech develop?'

'We just don't know,' replies Dr Schroeder. 'Some children at age three say a whole sentence when before they couldn't say a word.'

I just want her to speak any language at all. Polish. Sanskrit. A language composed entirely of swearwords. *Fuckbollocksarseprick*. It doesn't matter. I don't care. *Speak to me.*

I don't say this.

Instead, I bring up the matter of other syndromes. She confirms that many are linked to autism, and mentions one called Angelman's. I write the word in my notebook. According to the psychologist, children with the condition remain nonverbal all their lives, and can only communicate with sign language or computers.

'But we don't know if this is what she has, we're still putting together the puzzle pieces.'

I'm getting used to hearing this phrase by now.

Cognitive tests follow. Dr Schroeder opens a bulky black leather briefcase, gives Emily a football, wooden blocks, small sensory spheres to interact with. She's not interested, and wanders off to scratch the wall, dribble on her chin.

Her beautiful face. She's tired.

Outside the window, I register a low building, bare birch trees; frugal, late afternoon light.

Picture cards next. Dr Schroeder points to one of them.

'*Wo ist die katze?*' Where is the cat?

No response.

'*Wo ist Mama?*' Where is Mum? she says, extending her hand towards Anita. Emily doesn't follow.

She is given a jar with small Lego bricks to use as a shaker.

I glance up; notice a postcard on the wall. It bears one of those 'inspirational' memes: *Never, never, never give up.*

'She likes all instruments,' Anita says.

'Yes,' I say, seizing on this. 'She loves music. She can recognise a piece of music she's heard before.'

A tiny gold bell comes out. Its bright, plangent chimes fill the room.

Ting, ting, ting, ting.

Emily stands still, purses her lips, smiles.

Ooh, she cries.

Ooh!

It's clear Emily hasn't performed well. She will need to be retested, a module back: 16 to 24 months. These exercises were for her actual age group, 24 to 30 months. And next time Dr Schroeder will conduct the autism tests: more involved screening to assess communication and social interaction. She points to an ominously large black trunk under the desk.

We say our thank-yous and goodbyes, and I carry Emily to the car. As we drive away, we praise Dr Schroeder, but then there is silence. We cross the River Main, its oily currents visible. I watch a long barge make slow progress, tacking to avoid sandbanks. Then the endless, evenly spaced stands of silver birch start to fly past; and behind these, nothing but the darkness of the forest.

When we're back in the warm, bright flat, I play with Emily in the Wendy house. She's always happy in its one, cramped room, scrambling around on the carpet of coloured balls, throwing them this way and that, unearthing toys. But I feel numbed after the meeting, as if there is static, or fog in my brain. I can't process all that is happening. I have an urge to protect her; as if, as her father, it was within my power to stop everything, to keep her from harm, rescue her.

An odd thought occurs. If only she could stay in this room her whole life, and never go outside.

I Google Angelman syndrome. The first link to appear leads to a video of a three-year-old girl with the condition. I feel – what happens? A frozen sea opens within. The girl could be Emily. She had, and has, the same symptoms: early colic reflux, low muscle tone, Global Developmental Delay, and is nonverbal. Part of the clip shows her running, with tremulous legs, hands waving. It's how Emily runs.

The Wikipedia entry states the condition is often misdiagnosed as autism, yet, confusingly, one site calls it a 'syndromic form' of autism. Its most striking characteristic, apparently, is 'a constantly happy demeanour'. Angelman used to be known as 'happy doll' or 'happy puppet' syndrome. I flashback to the woman with the red scarf who stopped us in the street. *Puppe*, she said. Doll. Just like a doll.

There's more. 'Laughing in inappropriate situations' is another symptom. Well, that could define Emily. Also: 'very fond of looking at images of themselves'. I think of her staring at her own reflection in the mirror on the playmat, in Surbiton. The Beach Boys singing 'In My Room'. *Hello you, I find you strangely fascinating, oddly compelling*. Most sufferers develop epilepsy, and need lifelong, 24/7 care.

Later, as dusk is gathering outside the apartment, the lounge dim, lit only with candles, I pick Emily up and dance her around to Neil Young's 'Harvest Moon'. We waltz and we sway and suddenly I feel my throat closing up on the lines about still being in love, wanting to see you dance again. I don't want her to have Angelman syndrome. Please, please don't have Angelman syndrome.

The next day, in snowy conditions, I walk to the bridge over the *autobahn*. A moment from the psychologist's meeting has been disturbing me. When I told Dr Schroeder, proudly, how much I loved Emily's sense of humour, her happy laugh – which to my mind was slim proof of her normality – maybe she thought: *Angelman's*, and wrote it carefully in her notes with the blue fountain pen. Why else would she have mentioned it? I'm convinced now.

The snow stings my face, melts on my coat collar. I've been coming to the *autobahn* almost every day, to commune with it, to unravel my chaotic thoughts. There is something about the repetitive, unceasing flow of traffic as it fizzes and *smooshes* below, the long keening notes of high-sided vehicles, the sound of many tons of metal moving through space – the very air being displaced – that soothes the agitation in my mind.

Everything seems unreal, has the character of a nightmare. We're waiting with a Sword of Damocles above us: the genetics results, both ours and Emily's. If they reveal Angelman syndrome, I fear them with every fibre of my being.

The un-resting stream of vehicles continues below; cars, lorries, transporters, hurtling towards Düsseldorf or Hamburg, each with a yellow splash of light reflected before it on the icy tarmac. A river in motion.

This is my river now.

18

Once In A Lifetime

BEFORE LANGUAGE THERE was music. Thousands of years before speech evolved, the main form of social communication – the expression of needs and feelings – was extended vocalisation, or 'calls'. The principal ones were laughing – involving an exhalation of breath in a rhythmic fashion – and sobbing, involving an inhalation of breath in a similar manner. (The others were sighing, groaning; and crying or screaming, associated with fright or pain.) A theory, put forward by Terrence Deacon in *The Symbolic Species*, suggests that since these calls were symbolic communicators of feelings, it might be that melody – instinctive vocal utterances made up of various tones – preceded language in telegraphing emotions.

I've been reading again.

Music Therapy, Sensory Integration and the Autistic Child by Dorita S. Berger is my latest find. She ponders Deacon's theory that this ancestral relationship might explain why people seem pre-programmed to process music as symbolic of human experience. Why we can find a song sung in a foreign language as satisfying as one in our own. And why, ultimately, we can detect emotional meaning in the prosody, or inflection, of spoken words. The rise and fall of pitch, the variations of intensity, all transmit subtle meanings to the listener.

These ideas preoccupy me as I voyage deeper into the wintry, 'nonverbal' music of Cocteau Twins. Music where I don't recognise words, only states of mind, emotions.

One evening, at teatime, I sing a song for Emily as she sits in her high chair. Another original of mine, heavily in debt, once again, to 'Three Blind Mice'.

Knives, forks, spoons!
Knives, forks, spoons!

I take a clean piece of cutlery from the dishwasher, then hold it up for her to see before I put it back in the drawer, hoping she might make an association, and maybe pick up a word. I tell her it's called The Dishwasher Song. In A. Then I feed her dark, seeded bread with Gouda *Jung* and cherry tomatoes.

'Em,' I say, 'do you think you might like to speak to Daddy one day?'

She nibbles on a crust, flaps her hands, then bashes them down hard on the table, like a queen demanding silence.

'Are you just waiting for the right time?'

She stares out of the window, engrossed in a column of smoke rising up from behind the Norwegian spruce.

'Do you think you might want to share what's on your mind, sweetie?'

She takes a mouthful of food then turns away, as if lost in thought. As if she had learned to speak in a different life, and some distant echo memory had just returned for a fleeting second, strange news from another star.

*

It comes as a moving image, a waking dream. Not the childhood nightmare where I am in cold, fathomlessly deep water at night, here the sea is calm and warm. It is early evening and harbour lights are visible, yellow and orange, see-sawing gently up and down. I'm treading water with Emily – clutching her in the lifesaver's hold – one hand beneath her chin, our mouths just cresting the surface; taking in salty gulps of brine every now and again. I can hear our breathing, the muted swishing of our limbs. As I pedal my feet I take in the scattered stars above; a cuticle moon. I have no idea how we got here, or where Anita is – perhaps we're shipwrecked, or we're on holiday and went for a swim before dinner – but Emily doesn't seem distressed. She is a water baby, after all; we always used to say that when she was very little, splashing happily in the bath. *She's a water baby*. But something is worrying me. The ocean is pleasant and soothing, we don't seem to be in any danger, yet every time I look I notice the reassuring lights of dry land seem to be getting smaller and smaller. We are moving inexorably out to sea. Further and further out to sea.

I force myself to watch a series of 'red flags for autism' videos on YouTube, aware of the siege of emotions that will inevitably descend. All of Emily's symptoms are present in the children on show: the absence of interaction with others, the ritual behaviour, the lack of response to their name. One of the clips is a US news report on something called 'head lag'. It begins with the presenter blithely announcing, 'And now: the latest development in the battle against autism.'

The battle?

I find myself bridling at the notion that autism is something evil or shameful that needs to be battled against. This is potentially my daughter you're talking about.

I've never heard of head lag. According to the news report, 75 per cent of children with head lag develop autism. When you pull a baby up by both hands from a lying position, they allow their heads to 'lag' back as if they want to stare at the ceiling. Emily has always done this. She did it in the buggy back in Surbiton. She did it this morning as I carried her up the wooden staircase to the childminder. What's more, I raised it a year ago with the community paediatrician at Harefield House. She merely suggested it was linked to Emily's low muscle tone. Jane, too.

And now I feel angry again. Was there a conspiracy of silence? Interventions could have been made earlier if tight-lipped medical professionals had said, 'This looks like autism'. But then I'm reminded that the problem *is* medicine, or rather, science. 'Dr McNally is a medical man – and therefore a science man,' I said to Anita on the Christmas Day walk in Germany, a year ago. I think back to biology lessons at school. At the end of each experiment: 'conclusion'. No conclusion can be drawn until all the results of the experiment have been collated. But Emily's life is not an experiment.

I realise I must now do for Emily what I did for her when she couldn't crawl – exercises, but for the mind. Physiotherapy for the brain. Word books, puzzles, YouTube tutorials. Just sit her in the chair after the morning at the childminder's and slog through it, even though she will have little or no interest. A dim memory of an autism parent's comment on Mumsnet returns: 'It's hard, hard work, but you won't regret it.'

I put Emily's age-appropriate books away. *The Gruffalo, The Tiger Who Came to Tea, The Owl and the Pussycat*. Then I root out *Farm, Paddington's Word Book, Maisy's First 1000 Words*, a simple five-piece animal jigsaw, and we go to work. I put her in the high chair in the lounge so she can't escape, and set the puzzle in front of her on the table. I demonstrate first: 'Cat here. Fish here. Dog *here*.'

I hand her the pieces one by one. She throws them on the floor, then twists around in the chair, laughing, to see where they've landed. Then, with one sweep, the puzzle board is sent clattering on to the laminate. She laughs even harder. It's funny.

To her.

I start again. Put a grinning moggy in her hand.

'Cat *back*.'

I attempt to guide her fingers, loosely holding the piece, fitting it into the correct shape. She flings it away. We do this over and over again, until, after 15 minutes, I'm mentally exhausted.

I try the books next, repeating each word three times, gently turning her around when her attention wanders.

'Apple. Apple. *App-le.*'

Nothing. No interaction. It's as if I'm not even here.

I'm doing it all wrong. Watching a YouTube clip on autism therapies, an educator insists that you need to turn the usual teacher-pupil model on its head. Go *with* them – comment, interact with their play – and it will improve their social and communication skills. The idea is based on something called Son-Rise, a home-based play therapy system developed in the United States. Essentially, you monitor the child's behaviour until a cue for social interaction is shown. This means getting down on the floor with them, on their level, using 'parallel play' – imitating what they are doing. The core principle is: they choose the toy, they take the lead. Once you've gained the child's trust by capitalising on their motivation, the acquisition of new skills can begin.

Instead of sitting Emily in a chair I will shadow her movements around the room, leaving the books and puzzles that I tried to drum into her scattered in corners for her to find.

*

When I was 11 years old, in 1981, Talking Heads released 'Once In A Lifetime'. It was in the chart for weeks, and each Thursday, watching *Top of the Pops*, I would become engrossed once again by David Byrne's sweaty-lipped dancing in the fever dream of a video – and by the words to this curious song. I somehow knew they foretold my future; that I, too, would have a beautiful wife, and a beautiful place to live, yet wake up one day and not know where I was, or how I had got there. The future has arrived. I am in a strange country, living a strange life with a strange child, and I feel like I've never known less about a situation in my life.

Compounding the sense of dissociation in the lyric is the intimation of 'things behind', as Paul Nash put it. Water that runs underground. A suggestion of a mysterious river beneath our feet, tirelessly moving. This, and the song's unstable centre of gravity. Something very odd is going on rhythmically, as if two bands are playing at once, multiple competing accents that conspire to put the listener in a trance-like state.

I stumbled across the clip on YouTube and have been playing it every day. Emily loves it. She shrieks when she sees Byrne's flinching, spasmodic movements; the dances he adapted from indigenous tribes-people.

The second meeting with the psychologist, to run the autism tests. Dr Schroeder welcomes us into her office, as friendly as before, a smile in her pale blue eyes. At one end of the room is a video camera on a tripod. I take a seat in a corner; Emily – in a purple party dress this time – sits on the playmat with Anita.

Dr Schroeder drags the large black trunk from under the desk, opens it. The first toy is made of moulded plastic, and appropriate for a one-year-old. Press a button and a man in a hat pops up. We have the same one at home. The psychologist offers it to Emily, then quickly snatches it away.

'I'm trying to block play, to test her reactions,' she explains. 'Is there any look of protest or approval from her?'

Emily doesn't seem to mind.

Next she calls Emily's name. One, two, three, four times. No reaction. According to the psychologist, after the fourth time, and a physical prompt, the autism box is ticked.

A red football comes out. Dr Schroeder hands it to Emily, who immediately throws it on the floor. They repeat the action.

'Ka-boom!' the psychologist says each time.

Emily picks up the ball and starts to eat it. She notices me for a brief second; smiles.

Next: a blue and yellow water pistol that blows bubbles. Emily follows them as they float down, with sad eyes, and her characteristic flamenco hand movements, her Shirley Bassey shapes.

The gun whizzes. More bubbles.

Emily places her hands up in the air as if snowflakes are falling all around her. She emits a small cry. The last two bubbles, reflecting the harsh strip-lighting in the room, pop and are gone. I feel a pull of emotion in my chest. Memories of childhood scenes return. A photograph of my grandmother in our garden in Hitchin, blowing bubbles for my twin brother, 1970.

A blue balloon comes out of the trunk. Dr Schroeder blows it up, then lets it go. It flies across the room with a wet fart.

'*Und jetzt?*' she says. And now?

Emily doesn't react, doesn't follow the balloon with her eyes. Instead, she begins to make laps around Anita on the playmat with her fingers in her mouth. I watch her narrow back, her vulnerable shoulder blades beneath the purple dress.

The light outside the window is ebbing away. A winter's dusk. Those bare birch trees again.

Next: little yellow rocks that fire from a launcher.

'Another try where I don't give her what she wants,' Dr

Schroeder says. She clasps the toy in her fist. Emily reaches out, tries half-heartedly to prise open the psychologist's fingers, then gives up.

The test that follows is startling. A white sheet is placed over Emily's head. She stands motionless, like a small cartoon ghost. '*Wo ist Emily geblieben?*' says the psychologist. Where has Emily gone?

The sheet is removed, and she's offered a toy rabbit with wagging ears. She ignores it, runs to a corner table and upends a box full of colourful wooden blocks. I get up, cross the room, and put them all back. I can see our daughter is becoming restless. She makes a thwarted attempt to rip the tripod and camera over. Then she almost sweeps Dr Schroeder's papers off the desk, prevented only by swift parental reaction.

Outside the window the light has slipped away.

A large plastic toy bath is brought out. Inside is a doll – a 'baby' to bathe.

'*Wasche das Baby*,' says Dr Schroeder. Wash the baby.

Emily isn't interested. She wanders to a chair in a corner, raises a knee, ready to climb. She is barely interacting with the psychologist now.

Then there is a heart-stopping moment.

Dr Schroeder picks up the doll, gently wraps a blanket around its head, and in a sure, light voice sings Brahms's *Wiegenlied* – 'Lullaby' – the most popular German bedtime song for children. We had a series of hand-me-down toys back in England that played this melody. It sends shivers through me. So many nights spent trying to settle Emily in her cot were soundtracked by this tune.

Emily smiles, returns to the bath, climbs in, and starts stamping up and down like a grape-treader. Then she gets out and with one swift motion upends it. An even bigger smile on her face. She giggles. I feel the urge, too. It's hard not to laugh.

The birch trees darken against the dusk, becoming more solid in the foreground.

The tests appear to be never-ending. Next: a green plastic frog. At this point, I interrupt.

'Give to Daddy. Em, give to Daddy. I'll give it back – promise.'

She drops the toy without acknowledging me, then runs around in circles. I knew she wouldn't hand me the frog, I suppose I just wanted to demonstrate it for the doctor.

Seemingly random objects follow. A wooden pestle and mortar; a blue plastic cup.

'*Trinken!* Drink! Dr Schroeder pretends to sip from the cup. No response. Emily takes the cup, drops it onto the playmat.

The psychologist brings out two Tupperware containers: one containing pretzels, the other filled with wine gums. She holds a box in either hand.

'*Möchtest du Brezeln? Oder Gummy Bears?*'

Emily takes a pretzel; bites.

'*Lecker!*' says Dr Schroeder. Yummy!

Emily is smiling her beautiful secret smile now, the one that transmits she is pleased with the world, with herself. That everything is right. The one that gives me a surge of pure happiness in my heart. She runs around the room, brandishing the box of pretzels.

'*Bravo! Super gemacht!*' the psychologist says. Well done!

Finally, the tests are over. The camera is switched off. I'm slumped in my chair. The meeting has lasted one-and-a-half hours.

It's black outside now.

Dr Schroeder, perspiring lightly, returns to her seat behind the desk.

'If you're not sweating by the end, they told us during our training, you're not doing it right.'

It's clear Emily has performed poorly, despite 'a few things that were promising', according to the psychologist. She says she can't be 100 per cent sure it's autism, yet. I feel I should remind her we're still waiting on the genetic tests that might confirm it is something other than autism – including Angelman syndrome – but let her continue.

'When I was nodding did she imitate, was it intentional? When I was singing did she recognise the song? Or was it more down to her interest in music?'

I mention joint attention, did she notice any signs of it?

'She didn't caress or look at the doll. There was no reactive social smile. Normally, when there is an important adult in the room – the dad – they look for approval.'

Wearily, I mention that I did get a smile, but only once.

'She seems to get more from her mother,' she says, turning to Anita. 'You smile a lot for your daughter, like any sensitive mum. I saw Emily trying to start an interaction a few times, that is quite promising.'

The results will have to be complied and assessed, but it seems Emily's cognition is around 12 months. She has the 'mental age' of a one-year-old. And she's nearly two-and-a-half.

I bring up the question of the two languages – should I try

to speak German with Emily? I've been starting to think that raising her as bilingual is a huge mistake, with no speech at all at 27 months. Apparently, children make a 'neural commitment' to native language phonemes – the perceptually distinct units of sound in speech – and screen out others. They build words from these 40 or so sounds. But she doesn't have a single native language, she has two.

Dr Schroeder frowns, seems unsure. 'Only if both parents were fluent in each language,' she says. 'I would stick to speaking in English with her. Communication is more important.'

We rise, gather our belongings, book a follow-up appointment. Then we walk silently to the car park, Emily over my shoulder.

In the Polo, I notice Anita's eyes in the rear-view mirror, fathomlessly sad and tired. Eventually, she says, 'I don't think she has autism.'

'Well we better pray it is,' I say, instantly slipping into conflict mode – so easily done now – 'because the genetic syndromes are too scary to contemplate.'

We race through the night in silence. I hold Emily's hand as German songs play on the radio. We cross the River Main, hibernal blue in the dark.

When we arrive home, I carry Emily upstairs while Anita looks for a parking space. It's past our daughter's teatime. I set out bread, soft cheese, and sliced cucumber. Put some tunes on the iPod: *Jazz Standards, Volume 1*. 'Cheek To Cheek', 'In The Mood', 'Nancy With The Smiling Face'. I watch her open, happy grin after each mouthful, her eyes closed, her socked feet (tiny hearts today) resting on my knees. I tickle them to make her laugh.

Songs. Smiles. Joy. Love.

19

How To Bring A Blush To The Snow

FEBRUARY BRINGS A savage cold front from the east. A seemingly endless procession of blank, white days. I throw myself into singing for Emily, my own brand of amateur music therapy. With no word yet from the autism centre in Frankfurt, it's one of the few things I can do to help further her development.

If I can musical-ise a game or action, I do. I play her more and more guitar, introducing harmonic chords for the first time. These other-worldly, bell-like note-peels are produced by striking the strings with the plectrum in the right hand at exactly the same moment as the left-hand barre – over the fifth, seventh, or twelfth fret – is lifted. Think U2's early guitar sound. Emily approaches, watching eagerly. A smile appears. *What's this?* her eyes say. It's as if a switch has been thrown in her brain. She looks up, imaginary snowflakes falling around her.

I play long, arduous flamenco workouts: hitting the strings

with the heel or fingertips of my right hand while fretting a descending sequence with the left. A min – G – F – E. An Andalusian cadence. The gutsy sound rolls around the innards of the guitar. She's spellbound.

I learn and adapt a new music therapy song every day. 'Five Little Monkeys' grows a reggae undercarriage – *Natty Dread*-era Bob Marley. For 'Brown Bear', I place a capo up three frets. It sounds like a Jesus and Mary Chain tune, or 'The Book Of Love', by the Magnetic Fields. Then I speed it up to a chugging, gonzo Green Day punk song, and she laughs like a meerkat.

One day, searching the Internet while Anita works in another room, I find an article entitled, 'Why isn't everyone talking about music and autism?' The first line reads: 'kids with autism may process music in similar ways to typically developing children. In fact, it may be the only sensory input they do.' Intrigued, I read on.

The paragraphs that follow I consume with trembling excitement. I know instantly I will read them many more times. The writer claims that, early on, when the definitions of autism were unclear, a heightened response to music was on the list of symptoms. Later, music was seen to complement autistic children's cognitive tendencies, their proclivity for creating patterns. But most of all, it seemed to relieve frustration and anxiety, decrease their agitation, help them focus. Music appeared to improve their ability to master language, and made them better able to interact with their peers.

I knew I was on to something. A connection I've been groping towards in the dark has been made. If there's a link between music and language acquisition then it must be pursued. I ransack the Internet, reading anything I can find. Apparently, autistic children are ahead of their typically developing peers in telling the difference between two notes that are close in pitch. A remarkable percentage even have perfect pitch. Moreover, studies have shown that brain patterns of autistic and non-autistic people are markedly different listening to spoken words, but not when the same words are sung. And severely autistic children can even use music as a complex language that includes humour. It all makes sense – the peculiar integrity of Emily's expression when I speak to her: *why are you constantly making that strange noise?* Her little laugh as I play the funny lick in 'Wish You Were Here'. Her brain must be wired differently, in some mysterious way that I'm suddenly desperate to understand. I vow to learn more about the subject, but for the time being, the affirmation that her communication skills and social interaction – all but non-existent – might be improved by music therapy is enough.

I read one last piece, about an orchestra that visits special centres for learning disabled teenagers. The musical director speaks about how successful the interventions are, how excited the children become, how exposure to live music improves their concentration and social skills. He also says how moving the experiences can be, that often he finds his musicians afterwards, outside in their parked cars, crying.

A few days later, Emily is shambling around the living room as I attempt to tap out the *Abbey Road* drum solo on an empty biscuit tin. She stops, her back to me, and starts moving her hands like a conductor. Then she turns, comes up and presses her ear to the metal. I've always sung to her, but, increasingly, I've been using pure rhythm to establish a connection between us. Shakers, tambourines, hand bells – anything I can coax a solid 4/4 rhythm out of. Her response is instant, and always accompanied by the secret smile.

I place the tin to one side, and put on *Neu!'75,* the German band's third album. Then, sitting at the dining table, I drum along to the second track on side two, the steely, propulsive 'E-Musik', with the palms of my hands flat on my thighs. Fours, sometimes doubling to eighth notes. My toes jump on the floor like a coffee fiend. The song is sleek, repetitive driving music, perfect for the *autobahn.* There is only one riff, one chord – but there are two drummers, Hans Lampe and Thomas Dinger, who play the same stubborn, rigid pattern, no fills, only a double accent at the end of every second bar – *cha cha* – with machine-like tenacity. A heady, trance-like rhythm.

Emily wanders over and places one of her small palms on my moving right hand. Then she places her other one on top. Feeling the beat. I see it go straight through her; she has that expression again, the switch being thrown. Alternating current to direct current. She turns her face away, stares into the distance, makes an odd, whale-like noise.

Cooh.

She smiles.

Cooh!

The drumming soon takes on an unstoppable momentum.

Boom, crack; boom, crack; boom, crack – cha cha!

Boom, crack; boom, crack; boom, crack – cha cha!

A flanger on a low sweep strafes the track. Wagnerian cymbals clash. The song doesn't seem to want to end; it's passed the four-minute mark. My arms feel tired. What must the *drummers'* arms have felt like?

The rhythm is creating a spell. A magic circle in which Emily and I stand hypnotised. Pure *Motorik* pulse holds us captive, unvarying, unceasing, never peaking or leading to a crescendo, but plateau-ing, going in a straight line, going nowhere.

Boom, crack; boom, crack; boom, crack – cha cha!

Boom, crack; boom, crack; boom, crack – cha cha!

Finally, the track falls to a halt. A sound effect fades in – a strong wind with waves behind, a beach perhaps.

Emily is looking up at me, grinning.

The agonising wait for a definitive diagnosis (the results from the genetic tests are still to arrive) and for the autism centre in Frankfurt to contact us with a schedule of interventions continues. I turn to YouTube, a seemingly inexhaustible mine of 'information'. One day I stumble upon a documentary about an American couple with a young autistic son. The parents have been through all the familiar stages. Well-meaning friends saying, *oh, so-and-so didn't talk until they were three*; anger at paediatricians not mentioning autism sooner; the terrible feeling that every day ticking by without therapies in place is a day wasted; not 'enjoying' their child for a period of time; feeling exhausted at seeing everything they do with their little boy as 'a teaching moment'. They speak to camera, sitting side by side on a sofa, holding hands, finishing each other's sentences. Their faces are careworn yet their eyes seem eagerly hopeful of something. The husband says they see each other as 'teammates', and that he wouldn't have 'made it through' without his wife … I pause for a moment, and feel envy, mixed with something like trepidation. Anita and I are drifting further apart when we should be sticking closer together.

There's footage of the child taking part in his intensive therapies. He's shown a picture card of a cat. He understands what it represents, and utters the phoneme 'Ca'. A feeling of hopelessness descends. I just can't see Emily being able to do this, it would be an impossible feat for her. She would need to have the cognition available to link the two, and at the moment she simply doesn't. But then I felt like this with her mobility. Will speech be the same? Will a miracle occur? Maybe music is the key.

I read more online about autism, a miscellany of facts and conflicting opinions. Although, one thing that seems to be agreed upon unanimously is that no two autistic people will display exactly the same symptoms. 'If you've met one person with autism, you've met one person with autism,' is a phrase that appears a lot.

This peculiarity was first noticed in the 1940s when two doctors, an Austrian paediatrician, Hans Asperger, and an Austrian-American psychiatrist, Leo Kanner, discovered the condition independently of each other on opposite sides of the Atlantic. Kanner's boys (and they were mostly boys; autism is three times more likely in male children) were 'retarded', suffered seizures, and displayed a wide variety of repetitive movements: spinning, rocking, finger play, hand flapping; later given the collective term 'stimming', from 'self-stimulation'. There were often balance and co-ordination difficulties, and paradoxical sensory issues where some were intolerable (touch, loud noises) and some diminished (perception of pain). If there was speech it would often be formulaic or verbose, with flat intonation, or 'echolalic' – repeating another person's spoken words without an idea of their meaning.

Asperger's boys, on the other hand, had fewer neurological issues and were of extremely high, even superior intelligence – his 'little scientists' as he called them. It was as a result of this wide range of symptoms that English psychiatrist Lorna Wing, who had coined the term 'triad of impairment', later identified autism as a condition of 'considerable complexity': a spectrum. (Autism is now known as ASD – autism spectrum disorder.)

This bewildering variety of characteristics seems to be one of the reasons awareness of the condition is so poor. The general public need to be able to grasp something by a few easy signifiers. Lack of empathy, for instance. It turns out this is a myth – and a highly damaging one, leading to an idea of people with autism as aloof, cold, unable to feel. Nothing could be more inaccurate: their 'mind-blindness', or lack of a 'theory of mind' – being able to put oneself in another's shoes – doesn't automatically equal a lack of empathy (where the definition blurs with sympathy: compassion, concern). Indeed, some autists have a surfeit of empathy, just are unable to show it.

One thing that does continue to divide opinion is what causes ASD. In the 1960s, autism was thought to be an innate, inborn condition, a biological defect, sometimes confused with childhood schizophrenia. Another view held that poor parenting was responsible, that cold, remote 'refrigerator mothers', in an infamous phrase, were to blame. Gradually, this absurd notion was repudiated, and it was accepted that autism *did* indeed have a biological explanation, possibly genetic.

Then a theory that autism could be acquired gained ground. The sixties rubella epidemic was said to have produced children who later developed autism: kids who had been exposed to the virus prenatally, who began to develop typically, but then suffered a sudden loss of language or social behaviour around the age of two to four.

The notion of an acquired, regressive condition reached its peak during the so-called autism 'epidemic', an explosion of cases in the 1990s, and was linked to the MMR vaccine. The English doctor who suggested the causal relationship, Andrew Wakefield, has since been struck off, his paper utterly discredited, but suspicion in some parents still remains. Vaccination is a potent folk devil – incidence of autism has been increasing from one in 150 children born in 2000, to one in 68 today. So what is happening? Environmental factors? Genetics? An increase in diagnoses? A combination of all three? Nobody seems to know.

I read long into the night, my eyes dry from the screen, the snow falling in arcs outside.

I've been having strange, disturbing ideas. Bouts of magical thinking. Sometimes, when I can't sleep, I remember the doll given to Emily by the eccentric fortune-teller woman in Gran Canaria. 'A Princess for a princess'. Was it some sort of curse? I'm not a superstitious person, but in my present feverish state,

I fear I may have started to become one. When I dig out a photograph of the doll, I notice, with a jolt, that the flamenco pose it holds – hands above the head, fingers twisting – looks startlingly like one of Emily's Shirley Bassey shapes. Stereotypical gestures which I now know to be autistic stimming.

Another memory returns. One Sunday, in Surbiton, when Emily was about six months old, a pigeon found its way into the bedroom through an open window. It had shat everywhere, including over her cot (at the time, she was still sleeping in a side-crib attached to our bed). I found the poor bird perched on the curtain rail, afraid, regarding me with one orange eye. I called pest control, and a small, shifty fellow with a sparse beard that half-concealed a nasty glassing scar showed up at the front door. He insisted on being alone in the room as he released the pigeon to the wild, using a large beach towel. Anita and I listened outside the door as he did battle with the creature – a great clatter of wings followed by a curious silence. Then he sprayed the room with some sort of disinfectant, as their faeces, even the spore-carrying dust from their wings, can be harmful to children. On his way out, I recall he pointed up to the mezzanine and asked: 'Is that a loft? You got mice? I can sort out your mice.' Why have I remembered this? It's because, in some cultures, a bird flying into the house signifies death. And I'm wondering – seriously – whether this wasn't the moment our normal six-month-old disappeared, to be replaced by a changeling. An alien.

20

One Of These Things First

A FINE, SHARP, early spring day. The last of the snow has melted. The birds in the trees are talking to each other, excitedly acknowledging the ferment they can feel taking place.

Emily and I are on our way back from occupational therapy. I speak to her as I push the buggy, ask her if she liked the new therapist, if she had fun during the session; is she thirsty? I have always done this, and always will, regardless of whether she understands or answers. It puts me in mind of older people who say they talk to their deceased spouse each day. Or God. Her silence, like the Almighty's, is implacable.

I've started following some autism-related accounts on Twitter. Some post inspirational memes that are mawkish, but which nevertheless disclose hard truths, causing a burn of recognition. One reads: *For all the dads that have never heard their child say 'Daddy'.*

She needs intensive speech therapy immediately. My arms feel suddenly flu-ish when I think of how many words other children

Emily's age have. She needs trained professionals around her *now*. Her four hours of therapy a week are starting 'soon'.

I start singing her song:

Em-i-ly, cha-cha-cha,
Em-i-ly, cha-cha-cha,
We-love-you, cha-cha-cha,
Yes-we-do.

'Does it need another bit?' I ask, as if she's my songwriting partner. 'Does it need a middle-eight?'

I break into a run with the buggy, and try to imagine her side of the conversation. No, it's just fine. I will talk to her as if she can understand, even though from her there is only silence.

The meeting to discuss the cognitive and autism test results, with the neurologist and the developmental psychologist. We leave Emily with the childminder, and drive to the hospital, neither of us speaking. Despite the progress towards a diagnosis, things are at breaking point between Anita and I. We either argue or avoid each other, and I'm drinking more and more in the evenings to keep the depression and fear at bay.

There is drizzle, grey skies. Tyre spray; low visibility. The *autobahn* is busy at this early hour. With my new, superstitious eyes, I see omens in the trees. A single corvid – a rook or raven – makes a leaping ascent to the top of a bare, black alder.

Soon enough, the low buildings loom out of the mist.

We park the Polo, then wait outside Dr Maier's office.

Suddenly, they are here, with smiles, handshakes, small talk.

We follow them to Dr Schroeder's office.

She speaks first, summarising the findings from the cognitive tests: 'Emily's expressive and receptive language, fine motor skills and social skills are all at a level of 12 months, or lower. She has no other form of communication to assist with the lack of speech. On the plus side, her big motor skills are only a year behind.' The doctor shows us a graph. 'We will soon be able to diagnose Emily's condition as a disorder.'

'By what standards?' I ask.

'The ICD-10,' interjects Dr Maier. 'The International Classification of Diseases, published by the World Health Organization.'

I've been aware of her eyes upon us, rapidly switching from me to Anita, checking our reactions.

Dr Schroeder continues. 'It's only at age four to five that we will be able to tell whether her autism is high-functioning or not.'

The A-word. First mention here.

They are both considering us, cautiously.

'We did say this before, didn't we?' asks Dr Maier, 'that there is a high probability that autism is the disorder; that it might be coming.'

Anita and I are silent. I think of how far we have come since the first panic-filled meeting with Dr Maier last November, when autism was first broached.

Then Dr Schroeder speaks at length, with much sympathy in her voice: 'Make Emily feel appreciated, resourceful. Find out what works nonverbally. If she can feel that eye contact is valuable then she will learn to use it. Find out what she likes, let her rule the "conversation", let her lead. Her verbal modulation is actually good. Her consonants aren't monotone – this is a good sign. Her intonation is strong, varied.'

She moves to the autism test results.

'Emily didn't block, or look at the toys … her waving was stereotypical, not directed at a toy … there is developmental delay in all areas …'

Finally, she fixes Anita and I with a serious look.

'We highly suspect that autism is the reason.'

There is silence in the room.

Both doctors are staring at us expectantly, waiting for a reaction. They seem puzzled as to why we are mute, like seated statues. Perhaps this is where others have wailed and screamed in disbelief, torn at the carpet. Perhaps we don't look like parents who have just been told their only daughter has an all-pervasive, life-changing disability. I can't speak for Anita, but I have already accepted that Emily is autistic a long time ago. I am numb to it now.

'Yes,' continues Dr Schroeder, 'a high probability that there will be autism … in the years to come.'

They glance nervously at each other.

'There are no environmental factors,' Dr Schroeder goes on, 'nothing you could have done or could be doing better – it is her …' she searches for a word, 'her *disposition*. Keep on making her feel loved and important.' There is kindness in the psychologist's young, pale blue eyes. 'It's important to be in touch with her. Everything you're doing is right. She will profit just from hearing sounds …'

The appointment has overrun. The doctors become agitated.

Maier races through the genetic results: 'The "conspicuous" finding from the CGH was a fragile part of the chromosome, on 12 per cent of the cells, in location 2q13.'

2q13. I write it down.

'But there's nothing in the textbooks linking it to autism. There were no deletions or duplications found, either.'

But then, just as we're about to leave, a troubled-looking Dr Maier brings up Angelman syndrome. I feel a chill go through me. I was going to say something, but thought better of it. 'It's a maybe,' she says. *Maybe* Emily has it. But she's not sure – most of the children with the condition suffer seizures, and her EEG was fine. There may have to be further genetic tests.

And now I'm confused. I thought they *were* testing for Angelman's.

We conclude the appointment on this worrying note, the two doctors rushing off to their next meeting.

That night, I Google 'fragile 2q13'. A page of links to articles on developmental delay appears, one with a specific mention of autism. So why did Dr Maier say there was nothing in the textbooks that connected the two? The textbooks are out of date, then, as soon as they're written.

Folate sensitive fragile site on chromosome 2q13 was detected in a female proband with speech disorder and severe mental retardation. The same chromosomal aberration was also detected in her mother with normal phenotype ... fragile 2q13 was found in two cases out of twenty autistic children and in no cases out of twenty normal controls.

There is a microscope image of a chromosome, with arrows pointing to the breaks – the fragile sites. They resemble tiny pulled Christmas crackers.

I plunge into the online world of human molecular genetics. Lengthy, exhausting medical papers. It seems everyone has 'common' fragile sites, but a rare one can lead to severe problems.

Am I getting closer to the answer? Or did we voluntarily *pour* the autism into Emily, with the MMR? No, the theory has been discredited, and anyway, she had her vaccinations on the same day as the one-year developmental review. She was already far, far behind.

Real springtime is here. Walking with Emily in the buggy to occupational therapy, sunlight flickers through fences and juniper bushes. The air is warm, and buttercups dot vivid sections of grass as we head through the park. A blackbird swoops overhead. I start singing the Beatles' 'Blackbird' for Emily. Her hands twist; fingers flex. Greasy magpies hop, with heartless eyes.

'*One for sorrow, two for joy, three for a girl, four for a boy* ... Remember this?' I ask. 'We used to sing this, looking out of the bedroom window in Surbiton!'

Pink magnolia blossom blows silently around us.

Later, there is a play session in the apartment. I invent a raft of new games. Chasing wildly from room to room with the First Steps Baby Walker; lying on my back throwing and catching a football; knee-sliding on the large stuffed hedgehog, all the time remembering the Son-Rise program, following her lead. There is eye contact. And she laughs and laughs. Then, in the kitchen, she shows me she wants to be lifted up from the floor by her hands. I'm afraid I'll pull her arms out of their sockets, but she turns her smiling face up to me each time, never wants me to stop.

We even have a 'conversation'.

'*Ga!*' she says, and I match the sound:

'*Ga.*'

'*Ge!*'

'*Geh.*'

'*Ger.*'

'*Guh!*'

This is the communication the developmental psychologist spoke of. This is progress. This is breaking through to her.

Part III

Age two-and-a-half to three

21

After The Flood

Frankfurt, April 2017

FAST FORWARD. IT'S a month later, a Saturday in April. I'm making my way towards the city centre at two in the afternoon. I find a bar and order a Peters *kölsch*. *Groß*. Skiing is on the big screen, meaninglessly. I need a pen and paper to get some of the mental chaos down. The anger, sadness, astonishment, regret. My marriage to Anita is over. And today is the day – after one more dreadful, rancorous argument – that I know it is finally irretrievable.

I have to commune with my river, but not the road beneath the *autobahn* bridge: a real one.

Soon I'm in central Frankfurt. I cross Willy-Brandt-Platz, pass the imposing Opera House and head to a main road near the Jewish museum. I cross, and find myself walking fast through a large greened area – the Nizza Gärten – where students idly eat ice cream or drink beer on the grass. It's a warm spring day. I can smell it now: the Main.

I drop down a flight of stone steps and there it is, the broad flat sweep of the river. Its brown, turbid waters are fast-moving. Dirty foam sticks to the bank, part-concealing driftwood, cigarette packets, tin cans, empty vodka bottles. Moored pleasure boats, their guy ropes submerged, are bucked by the current. Hulls knock together, steel gangways creak in the sultry breeze.

She doesn't want any more of me. And I can't blame her. For the past year I've been impossible to be around, wrapped up in my own struggle, not once asking about hers. She will have been under immense pressure, too. Emily's ongoing diagnosis, the displacement of the move to another country, me being out of work; all of this – on top of the stress and strain found in any marriage; the challenges that face any two people in a relationship – has led to this final rupture. We should have talked more, argued less.

I walk and walk along the promenade, into the sun. Dazed, frightened. Everything meaningless: joggers, cyclists; two teenage lovers on a bench who stop kissing as I pass. A menu on a restaurant boat: *Bratkartoffeln und salat*, €9.80. Who cares? I'm not hungry.

Points of light dazzle on the water. Three long, low barges with mounds of sand glide by. A rowing boat follows in their slipstream; I watch as it is pulled out into the middle of the wide river.

Row, row, row your boat,
Gently down the stream,
Merrily, merrily, merrily, merrily,
Life is but a dream.

We were so happy. Or maybe it was just me that was happy.

The dream of a family, a trinity – a *completion*, really is over.

How long should I walk for? The path seems to stretch ahead for miles. My armpits are damp; I haven't showered. I notice steps that lead down to the water. Should I fill my pockets with stones? No: Emily.

I stand still in the centre of the path, bikes and runners flying past.

Wait. No. Stop.

This is madness. What the hell is happening?

I turn around and experience a lurch, like stepping onto a non-moving, out-of-order escalator. Couples with young children pass. Church bells boom in the distance.

I make my way slowly back.

When I return, the apartment is ringing with silence.

Three days later, I talk with Anita about me moving out. Costs, timeframes, vans. A terrible, surreal conversation. I put forward the plan I've been rehearsing in my mind: we move back to London, back where we started, co-parenting Emily in the same city. But only after she's four, maybe. There's no question of disrupting her existing therapies, or the autism interventions we're still waiting for here in Germany, they've taken months to set in place, and would take a similar amount of time, if not longer, back in the UK. By then, the window where 'all the learning machinery is constantly switched on' will have closed. No, she will stay here, while I return to England to find work. It's clear that staying in Germany is not an option for me: gigs are non-existent; I'm still unemployed.

I will visit Emily every few weeks. Then, when the time is right, I'll help find Anita find a job in London, arrange a flat, a car.

She doesn't dismiss the idea. But there is dread in my stomach. I know this is not how it goes in real life. I know, with a terrible feeling of sadness, that me moving out is the first step in losing my daughter.

*

I spend ten days in London. Late April. A dreadful, uncertain, heartbroken fortnight. My brother and sister-in-law kindly put me up in their house, while I search for a flat. But it is here, in this short span of time, that a Damascene conversion takes place. And it starts with a book.

I'm in Piccadilly Waterstones one morning, scouring the autism section for an up-to-date title, and after a fruitless 20 minutes, turn to leave. There, before me, on a display table is a weighty Penguin paperback with an attractive, colourful cover design featuring dozens of species of birds. It could almost be a Talk Talk album sleeve. Published the previous year, the book is called *In a Different Key: The Story of Autism*, by American authors John Donvan and Caren Zucker. Deciding there's much I like about it, not least the musical reference in the title, I bring it to the counter.

It takes the whole ten days to read, lingering over especially important passages. *In a Different Key* is a revelatory study, ranging from Kanner and Asperger to Lorna Wing, and Uta Frith – the psychologist who classified many of the condition's symptoms. From the benighted fifties and sixties, when parents were told to put their 'psychotic' children in institutions and forget about them, to the internecine wars of the US autism parents' movements of the 1970s, many of whom searched with evangelical fervour for a cure (there is no cure). From Ivar Lovaas, the professor who pioneered the controversial ABA – Applied Behaviour Analysis – therapy, to the labyrinthine investigations into the 1990s vaccine scare; all threaded through with personal testimonies from parents with autistic sons and daughters.

It's in these case studies that I learn more about the characteristics of autism – the deep need for order, patterns and repetition to counteract the frightening unpredictability of the outside world; the tantrums which aren't tantrums at all, but burnout caused by sensory overload, known as 'meltdowns'; the deficit of social instincts ...

I learn a new word: 'neurodiversity', a concept where neurological differences are respected as normal variations in the genome. From this comes the startling idea that I must *celebrate* Emily's condition. And it is a condition – part of her human condition. Not an illness, or a curse; she's not 'broken'. She doesn't need curing or mending, merely understanding. I now feel shame for talking about what is 'wrong' with her. There is nothing wrong, she is just wired differently to 'neurotypical' children, the term I use from now on instead of 'normal'. And I certainly don't regard her autism as a 'tragedy' any more. The fact that I used the word makes me cringe with embarrassment.

The origins of the neurodiversity movement can be traced to a Toronto autism conference in 1993, when a man with ASD named Jim Sinclair gave a speech to an audience of parents.

His phrase 'Don't mourn for us' was aimed at those mums and dads who mistakenly believed their autistic children had somehow been cursed by fate. Their message, Sinclair insisted, was clear – that autism was *bad*. Since the 1960s, the parents' movements and activists had formed organisations with names like Defeat Autism Now! or Cure Autism; books had titles such as *Targeting Autism*. Often the condition was depicted as an alien force or malign invader that had taken their children away. In 2007, an advertisement campaign in the form of a mock ransom note appeared on New York billboards: *We have your son. We will ensure he won't be able to interact socially or take care of himself for the rest of his life. This is just the beginning. Signed: Autism.* The resulting outrage from the neurodiversity movement ensured the campaign was scrapped within a month.

By the time I finish *In a Different Key*, the book has completely changed how I think about autism, about Emily, about life. Negatives have become positives. An illumination has occurred. In a curious way, it has given Emily an identity, a place in the world. And discovering neurodiversity – the concept and the movement – makes me feel less alone; that there might be thousands, possibly millions, of parents out there just like me. These are my people, I decide. My team. From here on, I have the zeal of a convert.

Throughout *In a Different Key*, names of other books are mentioned, the same titles appearing again and again. I decide to embark on an intensive, discriminative reading project. One of the books is called, rather ominously, *The Siege*. This will be the one I read next.

A second event makes me feel less alone. I spend an hour on the telephone with an autism parent, the first I've spoken to. Sally is a friend of my sister-in-law's, and has a ten-year-old autistic son.

It's a melancholy Easter afternoon, when, staring at the treetops and chimney pots of Belsize Park, I summon the courage to dial her number. She picks up promptly, and her first words are: 'Oh, we're just lying around on the sofa having a lazy Sunday!' This image of happy, relaxed normality arrests me. If it's possible for them, perhaps it is for us, too (although there is no 'us' anymore. I don't mention that my marriage has collapsed).

Throughout the call, Sally is friendly, enthusiastic, funny, understanding. The conversation ranges widely over Disability Living Allowance, supermarket meltdowns, diet, sleep, different therapies; and the fact that we're probably in the best era to have an autistic child. The sweet spot, post the terrible, institutionalised 1960s, and pre the inevitable day when the gene is found, and autistic people are screened out of humanity. We swap book recommendations, and I enthuse about *In a Different Key*. Most of all, we agree, there still isn't enough awareness of the condition.

She speaks warmly of her son. He hasn't been bullied at school, so far. More than once my throat closes up when she speaks of how kind and understanding his friends are. They look out for him, she says, on sports days, at school plays.

Then she says something unforgettable: 'One day your daughter will amaze you with what she can do; things you once thought utterly impossible.'

This isn't said lightly, I can tell. No experienced autism parent would offer false hope to one newly on the bewildering, painful road towards a diagnosis. She is impressed, too, that I seem to have accepted Emily's condition so quickly. It's all down to *In a Different Key*, I reply.

We agree to keep in touch, and, in the next days, I receive an email dotted with links to books and helpful websites. My gratitude knows no bounds. One of the titles, *Playing, Laughing and Learning with Children on the Autistic Spectrum*, by Julia Moor, I order straight away. *The Siege* will have to wait.

*

Back in Germany. Now Anita and I must try to get along in the apartment until a solution to where I'm going to live is found. Only being with our daughter has the power to lift my spirits.

One day, playing with her in the lounge, it strikes me that all the messing around I used to do with Emily as a break in the learning – the tickling, bouncing, chasing – was actually the learning itself. Or, at least, just as important. Once an autistic child sees that social interaction can be enjoyable, and thus valuable, in its own right, the fundamentals of communication can be taught. It's part of the theory behind the Son-Rise programme, and related to other interventions such as 'intensive interaction' and 'floortime'.

It's fortunate that Emily likes to be tickled. During our sessions, which are highly tactile, I realise she's been spared many of the sensory issues that come with autism. Yes, she has some, but plenty of autistic children, I discover, can't bear to be touched or bathed, even. Clothes can feel like fire on their skin.

Music first. This is always the key that unlocks the door to interaction. We start with tambourines (or rather, she does. I adhere to Son-Rise's first principle: let the child choose the toy). Soon we are bashing out rhythms. Then we do something I stumbled upon recently. When I peel the Velcro clasp on the lime-green hand tambourine slowly open, she giggles at the sound, moves closer; and steps into my orbit. She rarely does this of her own volition. I can't help but wonder if the music, the rhythm of the tambourines, contrived this somehow.

Next we embark on the intensive interaction. Or, to give it its technical name: fun. Since reading Julia Moor's *Playing, Laughing and Learning with Children on the Autistic Spectrum*, I've been finding it easier to play with Emily. The author comments that, at first, you may feel uncomfortable playing with an older child as you would with a baby, or a one-year-old. But you quickly forget this. And she's right.

We start with the Sellotape game. Soon Emily is chasing me, a twisted line of sticky tape between us, running wildly from room to room, both of us whooping and laughing. Then she will stop, and pull me. We take it in turns to lead. This is good. Whenever I feel my energy flagging, I spur myself on with a line from the book: 'games with rules are deeply social'. The line of Sellotape, like 'Wish You Were Here', is a cord of communication between us (and one that could easily lead to a visit to A&E).

For a break, we relocate to the kitchen to blow bubbles. The tube drips messily on the floor as I send flurries of oily, translucent, light-reflecting spheres jetting from the small plastic hoop. She considers them as they float around with great solemnity.

Finally, we use the mattress in the main bedroom as a trampoline. She climbs on, stretches her arms above her head; I hold her by the hands, and she starts to jump up and down. She giggles and screams, watching her hair leap in the mirrored cupboards adjacent. I count along. May as well get a teaching moment in.

One, two, three, four …

I can sense she wants to go higher, so I hold her under her arms, and on every fifth beat launch her high in the air with the word 'bounce'.

One, two, three, four – BOUNCE!

Each time she sees her head almost touch the ceiling she roars with laughter.

One, two, three, four – BOUNCE!

Then a quick round of roly-poly and tickling. I have to remove a metal coat hanger from the bed for this, and the sound of it clattering onto the floor sends her into hysterics. Eye contact!

Only when my arms start to burn, and I take her to the kitchen high chair does she protest. But it's a brief rebellion, and good, in a way. She's showing me that she wanted the game to continue: communication.

I've been brooding on a radio programme about autism that my brother sent me a link for. He warned me it was 'heavy'. It was. The two interviewees, a male author, and a woman named Christine, each have profoundly autistic sons who are now young adults. Because of the diminished quality of life the two men experience, both parents respectfully and carefully reject what they call the 'autism pride' movement – neurodiversity. I can see they have a point. Since my conversion to the cause, I've begun to realise that the autism community is deeply divided. In fact, it is less a community than a series of factions (another book on my list is Steve Silberman's aptly titled *NeuroTribes*). Their argument, in précis, is that a high-functioning autistic university graduate who can hold down a job, and perhaps even a relationship, is very different from an individual who can't speak, self-harms, and needs 24/7 care. Why, then, should all autism be 'celebrated'? With much emotion in her voice, Christine admits that, although it's been many years since her son's ASD diagnosis, she still wishes he didn't have one. She loves and is proud of her son, but if she could take away his autism she would.

I remain in the neurodiversity camp, but my zeal has cooled somewhat.

The author suggests there should be a new word for autism – or words, rather. An autism 'one', 'two', 'three', because of the huge variation in individual characteristics. Agreed. The more I learn about the condition the more I realise 'autism' is as meaningless as 'rock music'. There are too many sub-genres within the parent term.

Fears are voiced, which are my fears too. Christine is scared her boy, who is in residential care and needs constant supervision, will 'just disappear'. Although he has rudimentary speech, 'if he became ill, nobody would know, he would just lie in his bed and stop eating and drinking'.

The programme is almost impossible to listen to. But it does at least raise the issue of adult autism, which seems to be practically invisible. The focus always seems to be on the children – good for increasing awareness maybe, a cute kid is an easy sell, but autistic children become autistic adults. Where do they all go? This is something that will preoccupy me more and more in the weeks to come.

I finally find the nerve to read *The Siege*. The book was written by an American professor of English, Clara Claiborne Park, in 1967, and tells the story of how she successfully cultivated the social, intellectual and emotional development of her autistic daughter, while refusing to be discouraged at a time when autism was barely understood. She accomplished this via 'the siege' of the title – not an aggressive intervention, as I'd feared, but a gentle beguilement.

Early in the book, Park observed that her 20-month-old daughter, Jessy, lived in happy isolation, 'a solitary citadel', and unless she and her husband 'intruded, attacked, invaded', she would remain there forever, in self-absorbed nirvana. Park, a supremely self-aware writer, admits this was arrogant, as what did they think they had to offer? But her instinct, as a devoted mother, was to use every tactic she could find to entice, *seduce* Jessy out of her fortress. A siege born of love.

The first lines of the first chapter, 'The Changeling', send an electric current through me. 'We start with an image'. A small, golden child on hands and knees, circling around and around on the floor, contented, absorbed, not calling for the attention of her parents, not even seeing them. The child is 18 months old, an age for pointing, tasting, exploring, but she does none of these things. I think to myself what countless parents must have on reading these lines – that is *my* child. As I read further, I can see the accolades on the cover are justified – 'classic ... timeless ... a must-read for anyone who wants to understand autism'.

The book also confirms that I've been stumbling in the dark, conducting my own instinctive siege with Emily – the games, and, most of all, the music.

22

New Grass

ONE OF EMILY'S hand gestures gives me a start. It reminds
me of someone. Who? Philip Bennett, a frail, sensitive, sickly
child who was mercilessly bullied at my all-boys' secondary
school. His nickname was 'Philys'. I wonder if he was autistic.
The many torments he suffered – the worst of which were
perpetrated by the teachers – come trickling back. I remember,
once, watching Bennett picking at a hole in brickwork as the
class queued outside the Geography block. His deep absorption
in the task, his odd finger movements, fascinated me. The
teacher breezed along the line and smashed Bennett in the back
of the head with a textbook. His skull connected with the wall.

Bennett held pariah status because he was different, *weak*.
And that was what really enraged the teachers, many of whom
taught sports or PE as a side subject – he was 'a weakling'.
What's more, he passively accepted his daily ordeal, never
answered back. In fact, I cannot remember him ever speaking.
The most shocking episode was when our form teacher led a

chant of *Phil-ys*, *Phil-ys*, *Phil-ys* as we sat at our desks. I recall the bumptious look on the man's face – just a bit of harmless fun – and Bennett cringing, cowering, being destroyed.

The pupils treated him almost as badly. 'Retard', 'Spazz', 'Freak', 'Mong' were his other nicknames. I don't believe he had a single friend.

The thought of Emily being bullied and ostracised in this way stirs primitive emotions. I cleave to the fact that she is tall for her age, and despite her low muscle tone, strong. Wilful, too. The way she bats the cup or spoon away when she doesn't want any more water or food is encouraging. She's going to need physical strength to survive in life.

But none of this brings much consolation. I don't sleep well the night after the memory of Philip Bennett returns. It consumes me for hour after hour. I think, too, of something Christine said on the radio show. When her autistic son was being bullied at school, he came home one day and asked for a Harry Potter invisibility cape, so the others couldn't see him, and the torments would stop.

I just have to hope what Sally said is true, that children, if they become used to someone who is different early on, behave with compassion and decency.

A few days later, an astonishing breakthrough occurs. At the end of our intensive interaction session, Emily and I are sitting on the playmat. I'm trying to persuade her to drop a blue tactile ball into my hands. Several times it nearly works, but I sense she doesn't really comprehend the task. As she loses interest, and starts to crawl away, I ask: 'Shall we go and bounce?'

She stops moving, starts smiling. Then she raises herself up, reaches for my hand and leads me along the corridor to the main bedroom.

'Oh my God, you understand!' I say.

I can't believe it. She locates the correct door, pushes through, hooks her right foot up onto the mattress and raises her arms above her head. She's already attempting to jump up and down as I take hold of her hands.

But as she leaps higher and higher, her laughter ringing around the room, a misgiving occurs. We've been here before, haven't we? When she clapped her hands, in the kitchen in Surbiton, a year ago. But this is different. She understood the *meaning* of my phrase, or at least recognised the word 'bounce'. I'm sure of it. This is her first ever sign of basic cognition.

We shall see. If it happens again tomorrow, I'll know for certain.

It happens again. The next day, she *does* respond to 'Shall we go and bounce?' Her back is turned, a smile forms, and she reaches for my hand.

Afterwards, I take her for a walk. It's a balmy, sun-dipped May morning, and I'm exalted at this new development. It recalls a moment in *The Siege* where, during a drawing session, Jessy leads her mother to the room where a pencil sharpener is. 'If she knows this,' Park writes, 'what else does she know?' In another book I'm concurrently reading, Charlotte Moore's exquisitely observed, clear-eyed account of bringing up two profoundly autistic boys, *George and Sam*, I learn that this is something familiar to many autism parents. She claims her sons understand far more than they show. It simply doesn't occur to an autistic child to share their knowledge, she writes, as they lack this basic social instinct.

In *George and Sam*, I also discover that bouncing on trampolines is a well-known autistic enthusiasm. It turns out one of her sons is a champion. Later still, I read online that there is a 'learning window' at the peak of the bounce, when the child's head is at its highest. It's where I say the word 'bounce!' So maybe that's how the connection was made? Curiouser and curiouser. The more I investigate, the more I discover.

'*Warum?*' asks the little girl sitting on her dad's shoulders. Why?
Then a word I don't understand, from the father …
'*Deshalb singen vogel?*' she asks. So that's why birds sing?
'*Genau*,' says her dad. Exactly.
I'm on my way back from the childminder when I find myself falling into step behind a tall young man and his daughter. As I pass them I try to tune in to their conversation. More words that are indecipherable, then:
'*Was ist das, Papa?*'
'*Eine kirche.*' A church.
We're passing a building that looks like a youth club – the modernist church. He's teaching her the world. I feel the old pain, but it passes quickly. I'm beyond that stage now, of what has been 'lost'. I'm aware only of what has been gained, the advances Emily seems to be making; the scrap of cognition around the word 'bounce', at an age when most children would understand, and be using, hundreds of words. 'There is no failure in autism' is another phrase that appears a lot. What

it means, I think, is every piece of progress, however small, is an unqualified success.

Emily will be starting pre-school soon. After much searching, Anita has found a rare place at an *Integrativ* kindergarten, a 20-minute drive away. This is an immense stroke of good fortune – Emily would be killing time for another year with the childminder otherwise, not learning much, and not socialising with other children.

But this coup brings its own worries. It's not the scrutiny of parents that concerns me now, it's that of Emily's contemporaries. One day, pushing Emily in the buggy, we pass a local nursery. I notice a little girl with her fingers hooked through the fence. She can't be older than three. The way she coolly evaluates Emily, who is dribbling, twisting her hands, I know she senses there is something not quite right. I can see it in her eyes: the keen, animal intelligence has picked it up, sniffed it out.

Later that day, returning from the childminder's, we pass the same spot. I watch Emily's hands flex at the wrist as she responds to the stimuli around her, the faint early summer noises: the rustle of leaves, a plane far off, the distant clamour of children. She tips forward in her buggy, staring at the moving pavement as if leaning over the side of a riverboat, watching the water as it gushes beneath the hull. The gentle breeze ruffles the flaxen hair on the back of her head, the down on her sweet, vulnerable neck. What will her first day be like? I ask myself, walking with the pushchair, no sounds now besides the squeak of the wheels and the *smoosh* of the wind in the trees. The kindergarten group she is about to join has a broad age range, two to six. It will be very different from the one in Surbiton.

A little girl flashes past on a tricycle, sending Emily the same suspicious look as the child behind the fence did.

What will it be like for her?

May is transforming the suburb. Sight lines are blocked by rapidly growing foliage. I go running in the park, Talk Talk's *Laughing Stock* on the iPod. Sheaves of *Maeinshein* – 'May-light' – drop through the trees, like an underwater scene. A motorised lawnmower manned by a *Stadt* employee executes sweeping turns nearby, throwing sweet-smelling fresh-cut grass in the air. All around, Frankfurt is in bloom: undeniably ravishing. But there is a bitter taste in my mouth. Soon I will be leaving.

'New Grass' comes on. The two-note guitar figure first, a fanfare announcing the arrival of spring, so longed for on the previous record. Then the piano chords in the bridge: glowing points of light like fireflies, just behind the beat …

So what was Mark Hollis searching for, in Wessex's studio one, recording *Spirit of Eden* in 1987? The answer, I think, was silence. Talk Talk's music at this point alternated between passages of near silence – in which the ambient sound of the room is heard, or *felt* – and startling explosions of sound. These sudden moments of violence stir powerful emotions in the listener, but so do the silences. They are not 'intermissions' in the jazz sense, a hiatus in the music, but the music itself. Silence always seems to be where the song is heading, its destination.

In Hollis' voice, too, the impulse towards silence can be detected. It still retained the natural power used so effectively when Talk Talk had been a pop band (I recall, aged 17, witnessing their final gig at the Hammersmith Odeon, his voice the loudest instrument, mixed so high it caused the balcony to vibrate), but increasingly it was becoming a whisper, an aching murmur that communicated emotion without using recognisable words. Oblique, yet desperate to connect.

And in the few words that *were* intelligible, a quest for spiritual sanctuary, a respite from the clamour of the temporal world, was palpable. A desire for an integration of thought and sensory experience, a *simplification* of life, described in Buddhist texts. Silence as a place where one is receptive, not active; able to understand the world afresh.

Ten years after the sessions for *Spirit of Eden*, in an interview to promote his first, eponymous solo album, Hollis admitted that silence was becoming ever more important to him. He listened to music less and less. *Mark Hollis* was also his last solo album. After the record's release he was publicly silent, producing no more new material, as if he'd said all he had to say ...

The trees throw glades of deep shadow across the park. On a steep verge, implausibly green in colour, I circumnavigate a group of students with their rucksacks and bikes. They're smoking something pungent.

New grass.

23

I Believe In You

'EASY CONCEPTION?' ASKS the doctor.

'Yes,' I reply.

'Any other children?'

'No.'

'You're 48, right?'

And here he grins irksomely.

'Yes, I am.'

We're in Central Frankfurt, with Emily. A meeting with the geneticist to discuss the latest findings.

Dr Lehmann is in his early thirties. Designer stubble, expensive frames. Very much the high-earning German professional. He likes grey: grey Lacoste polo top, dove-grey chinos, grey leather Camper shoes. It's a slightly effete look, yet it's clear he's a 'macho', as they say here – asking cavalier questions, then talking over my answers.

His room is wide, wood-floored. There is a balcony, with decking, a rose plant, and a view over the top of a horse chestnut tree into central Frankfurt. The sky is gauzy; a sleepy European summer is beginning.

Emily, in a print dress, wanders off to explore the space, crawling on the floor, eating the soil in the pot plant, straying worryingly close to the plug sockets, until Anita pulls her away.

After a few more preliminary questions, we plunge into the meaning of the fragile site on chromosome 2q13.

'It *could* be the reason for your daughter's disorder,' ventures Dr Lehmann, 'but we don't know. It can't be proven. There's no test available to confirm that it's pathogenic.'

Apparently, the chromosome isn't broken, merely stretched so the spiral ropes become almost invisible.

I bring up autism.

He regards me neutrally.

'In ASD, genetics only accounts for 10 to 20 per cent of cases,' he says.

I would have mentioned the A-word earlier, but because of his domineering manner I've been cautious. He embarks on a monologue about the breadth of the condition: 'I used to have a boss next door that would email when he could have talked to me, was he autistic?'

Yes, yes, I know, I want to say. Instead, I utter a few phrases that show I've read around the subject. Something new enters the way he looks at me.

Then Angelman syndrome is broached. He says they will investigate the relevant chromosome, number 15, seeing as the neurologist has voiced a concern, and because we're worried, too.

Next, Dr Lehmann sits Emily on a small plastic stool to conduct a physical examination. Reflexes, lungs, eyes … I have little enmity for the man now; he's gentle with her, attempts to communicate. I wonder if he has kids of his own, a question I always ask myself about the doctors.

But then he finds something unusual about her head measurement.

'2mm … it could be an error. But it could also be a hint.'

Sweat bubbles up under my skin.

'A hint for what?' I ask.

'Rett syndrome.'

I try to recall if I've come across this in my research. It's when the child stops developing, isn't it? The head stops growing.

'If it's Rett's,' he continues, 'the prognosis isn't good.'

I glance at Anita, her face in three-quarter profile; there are tears in her eyes, just threatening to brim over her lower eyelids.

'Is it more common in girls?' I ask.

'Yes, *only* in girls,' he says, sending me a severe look. 'In boys, the genetic error is fatal.'

'Can we have her tested?'

'In genetics, if you have an idea, go for it …'

Lehmann pauses, seems to reconsider, then says, 'Yes, do it – but of course, I hope it's not true.'

He returns to his desk and consults Emily's notes on his screen. As he scrolls down he says, 'And you know there is a 10 per cent chance of autism occurring in a second child.'

Of course. The only reason he's giving us so much of his time is the assumption that we may be planning for another baby.

I don't answer.

Still squinting at his monitor, Lehmann says, 'Parents are more ambitious than doctors about Internet research …'

I'm expecting the attack on me now – the desperate, unqualified father with his ragbag of Google 'knowledge' – but he's smiling playfully. 'So if you see anything on 2q13 …'

I can't believe it.

I tell him about my simplest of searches. He types it in.

'Ah, yes. Here it is. Kyoto, 1992.'

The little girl with the fragile site on chromosome 2q13.

He skim-reads it, then says: 'But it's only one paper.'

I remind him about the autism mention.

'Yes,' he says, 'it's a self-fulfilling prophecy, because the CGH is only done if autism is suspected. It's a very expensive test, you know.'

We seem to have reached some sort of impasse. There is a consent form to sign for the Rett syndrome screening (not because of harm to the child, but the psychological consequences for the parents). Then we make our way to the lift. Outside, the hot, sticky streets are dense with people. Anita buys an ice cream for Emily, then we each take one of her wrists and walk her, me trying to push the empty buggy through the crowds with my free hand. I study her dirty, cherubic face as she concentrates on the human traffic. I try to remain calm, and assimilate what we've just heard. So there are three hats in the ring now. Autism, Angelman's – and Rett's.

The next day, I'm feeding Emily porridge with raspberries for breakfast, *Revolver* by the Beatles playing. She breaks into a smile when she hears the sitar intro to 'Love You To'. That first jubilant, cascading peel of notes, played by a backwards fingerstroke. Then, as the musician explores the chord, picking out melancholy arpeggios on the traditional Hindustani instrument, Emily's eyes change, become distant and sad, yet her smile remains frozen. She seems to know the music is conveying something else. There is indecision in the sound. Finally, the great eight-note fanfare arrives, the tune surges into life with drums and bass, and her eyes change again: *Yeah!*

Sensing she's in a Beatles mood, I clear the breakfast away and we move to the sofa in the lounge. I begin 'Ticket To Ride' on the acoustic, but the instrument is out of tune. As I remedy this, she bashes the body of the guitar in order to hear the different variations of tones, the hollow ring of its interior. Then she clambers up next to me and tries to climb *into* the guitar. I persevere, watching her consider how a pick stroke near the bridge produces a more callow note to one nearer the sound-hole. She holds the strings down with flat palms, muting them, to experience the vibrations.

'Bear,' I say, 'I'm trying to tune up here. You know I care for your ears,' a reference to the live album, *Hendrix in the West*, that will be lost on her, but which I say anyway.

Before we start I turn the guitar over so she can see her reflection in its glossy, lacquered back. She laughs when I tilt it so it distorts her, an image in a fairground mirror. Then I flip the instrument around, and run the pick down the serrated, wound low-E string to make a heavy metal screech. She makes rapid thumb and forefinger movements, like flicking peas; forms her lips into a pout, a lead guitarist's solo face.

Then I play the song. The bright, chiming notes of the opening riff enchant her. She places her hands flat on the soundboard, and turns her face away in radical concentration, remaining like this for the rest of the tune.

As the last echoes of 'Ticket To Ride' ring around the room, I apologise for – and attempt a context explanation of – the chauvinism in Lennon's middle-eight lyric, then place the guitar back in its case.

Next, I sing 'Sgt. Pepper's Lonely Hearts Club Band (Reprise)' for her, accompanied by just a shaker. I lie on the rug, and she climbs up onto my chest. She knows the routine by now. Four-bar intro – Ringo's drum pattern on human beatbox, then the count-in: Paul's buoyant, assertive *One-two-three-four!*

I do the guitars for her next: *Drang, drang, drang, drang!*

And we're into the vocal.

I've started in too high a key, but never mind. Emily grins in recognition as each verse unfolds. She reaches out, tries to take the shaker from me. I tighten my grip. She's making noises, 'singing' along.

I negotiate the key change, but am tripped up by the additional *one and only* Lonely Hearts Club Band. It goes against the grain, as it were; one of the countless, pleasing touches of genius the Beatles put on their albums. Emily doesn't seem to notice. Her delight in the song is unwavering.

I hit the extended notes of the coda, and end in a flourish on the shaker, held high above our heads. The last '*Whoo!*' that is on the record. A trash-can ending.

There is wan disappointment in her eyes. She can't say 'more' but I know that's what she wants. Her weight on my chest is becoming uncomfortable. I promise I'll do 'A Day In The Life' for her tomorrow.

*

Two weeks later, I'm in a pub on Haverstock Hill. A video of Emily sitting on a yellow plastic swing is playing on my phone. She is dressed all in purple, hair held back in matching clips, her ginning face zooming into the camera, then zooming out again. Back and forth, a compelling motion, like speeded-up film of waves on a beach. Beneath her, on white paving stones, sun-dappled shadows play in a rectangle of sunlight.

This is all I have of her for now, a precious fragment. Forty-one seconds of her. I play it over and over: the frame freezes, I tap the circled arrow again. As she reaches higher and higher, the swing starts to judder; she begins to giggle, tries to turn around in the seat, her hands twisting, flexing, waving. She looks down and notices the shadows on the patch of sunlight rushing below her and the giggles turn to bubbling laughter.

How she loves being alive. I want her to stay this happy forever. I'm envious of the delight she takes in the moment, as if she has discovered the meaning of life without even trying. The phrase that came to me in Long Ditton rec, Surbiton, the first time she sat on a swing returns: *You can have a bit of everything, my darling. Think of life as a feast – you can have a bit of everything.*

I press 'play' again and stare at the girl in the swing. Her hypnotic movement, her untiring joy. I'm crying so hard I can barely see the screen.

Sultry June rolls on. I'm back in the top room of my brother and sister-in-law's house in north London while I search for flats.

It's proving far harder than I thought it would be, regaining a foothold in the capital. I might have to look further afield: Surbiton, maybe.

One day I find myself in a cafe, listening to the voices of a Saturday dad and his young son sitting behind me. I noticed them on the way in – the boy, wearing a lime green T-shirt, blue shorts, had something odd about his eyes. He's making hoarse vocalisms now, the father becoming agitated. Something, a glass of orange juice maybe, must have been knocked over.

'Max, it will dry.'

'It won't dry.'

'It *will* dry.'

'It *won't*.'

Could he be … autistic? Abruptly, the boy shoots past me to the door, and it's confirmed. He stops, clasps his left hand to his forehead like a tragic actor, his right dangling by his side. The fingers curl, stretch, make the characteristic shapes.

I have a powerful urge to make contact with the dad, but what would I say? I want to offer support, kinship; and to feel that returned. I want to speak to someone who understands what I'm experiencing. Someone further into it than me, with wisdom and advice to give. I say nothing, and feel alone as I watch the child run back to the table.

From here on, I see them everywhere, the different ones, the autistic boys and girls with their stereotypical gestures and noise-reducing headphones. I smile at them, feel close to them; they are Emily's brothers and sisters.

*

Germany. Late June. My last day in the apartment. I bequeath Emily my guitar – the old Suzuki acoustic, the instrument I wrote all my songs on in my twenties – in the blind hope she will be able to play it one day. Sally's words return: *Your daughter will amaze you with what she can do; things you once thought utterly impossible.* I need to clean it up for her, the strings are old now, black filth comes off on my fingers. The sound-hole of the guitar, which Emily peers into as if it's a cave, or the mouth of a volcano, reveals a blood-spattered interior from fingers flayed in a thousand smoky pubs and subways. I put it back in its battered hard case – the one that lay open on Westminster pier where I busked as a 21-year old – and place it carefully on top of the wardrobe in the bedroom. Ready for my first return visit.

Then I change and dress Emily; brush her hair. I kiss her head, and tell her Daddy's leaving, but he's coming back. He will always come back. And I feel tears prickling in the bridge of my nose, like the onset of hayfever. I leave my keys on the side, by the microwave; and my heart, crushed into a thousand pieces.

24

In My Room II

'HOW ARE *YOU?*' asks the beaming woman. 'More importantly, how is *Germany?*'

Back in Surbiton, emerging from the station, the first person I see is Anna, our downstairs neighbour from the old flat.

I tell her about Emily first. The smile drops. She looks around, as if searching for someone.

'No, but ... autistic? I can't believe it.'

Then I inform her that my marriage to Anita 'didn't last'. I have to be careful about how much I reveal; there will be more exchanges like this. The NCTs still live in Surbiton. Tim and Cassandra. People fear failure; it might be contagious. The whole thing sounds like some hard luck story, a bad Country & Western song: my kid got a diagnosis, then my marriage imploded. What next – a tornado takes my house and car?

Don't tempt the gods.

I tell her that Anita and Emily will be coming back to Surbiton, although I don't say this is far from certain, and possibly my own wishful thinking. Anna is sweet, understanding; offers useful information. She tells me a nearby school has an autism unit. I didn't know that, I say. Maybe we were in the right place all along. I show her a picture of Emily on my phone. She gasps when the smiling, impossibly beautiful face appears on the screen.

'She's a happy little girl,' I say.

I'm eager to emphasise that this isn't a tragedy.

Emily isn't a tragedy.

She wishes me luck, and we say our goodbyes.

I am starting my new life in the old town, returning to the precarious margins, the minimum-wage job.

The flat I eventually find is in a 1990s block on the border with Surbiton and Long Ditton. There are the inevitable stale carpets and sticky door handles on the kitchen cupboards. Landlord magnolia on the walls. Tacky, imitation gold lamps in the lounge, a fanciful suggestion of luxury. Only Saddam Hussein had this much gold in his house, and at least his was real. I hang my modest collection of hats on them. The rooms are hired boxes for office workers, retirees, divorcees … Subconsciously, I think I chose the location so that I could be near to the places where I spent time with Emily: Long Ditton rec is visible from the lounge window, I can hear the trains as they charge past at the far end, trailing their ghost notes. Each morning my thoughts turn to her, and what she is doing in Germany. Is she happy? Sad? Eating? Playing? Pooing? I'm separated from the most important person in my life.

For much of this period, although I don't realise it, I'm

in a kind of long-range shock. I create a cave in the living room, a retreat made from cushions and blankets, and from here, comfort-watch some of my favourite childhood films. A cineaste's version of listening only to the old music. And in these movies I find something I didn't expect: autism.

The first DVD I load into the cheap, newly purchased player is *Close Encounters of the Third Kind*. My father took my brother and I to see it in Paris, where he was working at the time. It was 1978; I was ten. The film had a huge impact on me – the special effects were mind-blowing, but I also suspect the subplot of family breakdown had resonance, too. It was the year my parents finally separated.

The little boy – Barry – who is kidnapped by the alien mother ship is 'different'. He has classic autistic traits: he's nonverbal, has no fear, runs away laughing from his mom when she calls his name. The scene in which he is snatched from their remote mid-western home at night is still terrifying. We never see the mother ship. Instead, an unseen force menaces the house, swamping it with a nauseous, overpoweringly bright orange light, until the boy is sucked helplessly through the kitchen cat flap, his distraught mother screaming '*Ba-ree!*' after him.

What strikes me about this scene, what it immediately makes me think of, are those ransom-note billboards: *We have your son. This is just the beginning. Signed: Autism.* It is the idea of ASD as kidnapper – a mysterious outside presence or malign invader that has the power to spirit children away – made explicit. I now know from reading *In a Different Key* and other books that the idea of a 'stolen child' replaced by an alien has long been a trope for autism parents. (Indeed, the first chapter of *The Siege* is called 'The Changeling'.)

But what I find really interesting about *Close Encounters* is the attempt to communicate with the aliens is made via music – the famous, repetitive five-note phrase. Towards the end of the movie, as the mother ship hovers over the military base on Devils Tower, the humans play this simple tune over and over again, trying to 'talk' to the aliens. The mother ship plays it back, at deafening volume, shattering all the windows, and a nonverbal discussion using music ensues. Finally, after physical contact has been made, the beautiful, silent alien queen walks up the ramp to the mother ship, and the credits roll.

I look up *Close Encounters* on Wikipedia. Apparently, an early draft of Steven Spielberg's screenplay featured an autistic boy 'cured' by aliens at the end.

Each night I watch a different film from my youth. In *The Man Who Fell to Earth*, David Bowie plays Newton, 'The Visitor' from another planet, and the perfect analogue of an autistic child-man. He doesn't understand that he has to shake hands in greeting, misses the point of questions, is disorientated in shops, doesn't comprehend money, is overly sensitive to light and noise ('The trains sound so strange here'). He becomes involved with a woman, Mary-Lou, played by Candy Clark, but she soon finds him impossible to relate to. She calls him 'simple', an alien, yells: 'You don't know how we live here.' Relenting, she says, 'You must hate me'. Newton replies he doesn't hate anyone: 'I can't.' In the climactic reveal, when Mary-Lou opens the bathroom door to discover Newton as he really is – lizard eyes, no brows; a creature from outer space –

her shocked, disgusted reaction symbolises society's revulsion with 'others', with autism.

In *Equus*, the strange boy (Alan Strang), whom I always assumed suffered from schizophrenia when I watched it on television as a teenager, is swiftly revealed to be autistic. In an early interview with the psychiatrist, portrayed by Richard Burton, he reels off snippets of *Typhoo* TV adverts – echolalia. His walk is childlike, his expression vacant or confused, mouth open; his utterances literal or inappropriate.

In *The Apartment*'s first scene, socially awkward C.C. 'Bud' Baxter, played by Jack Lemmon, is obsessively calculating how many employees work in his office ... I reach wearily for the notebook again: Asperger's.

In *Tommy* ...

Even films that are just intrinsically strange, such as Wim Wenders' German- language *Wings of Desire*, there are minor characters with autistic traits. The little boy who is ostracised by his friends, who says he's all alone, 'just mad on my own'; the disabled girl in glasses who wonders if life under the sun isn't just a dream. These speech fragments are overheard by Bruno Ganz, playing an angel who has the ability to tune into people's inner dialogue. Only he and his associates – his fellow angels – have the power to hear what others are thinking in silence, to commune with these separate selves as they move through time. They perceive the 'things behind', '*Der Welt hinter der Welt*' – the world behind the world.

I ponder why there were so many autistic characters in films back in the seventies and eighties. Yet they were never labelled as such. I think of Richard, too, the disabled boy, my father's partner's child. I can't help but wonder if he may have been autistic. In my current state of magical thinking, it feels as if autism has been stalking me since childhood. My dad's apartment in Paris was opposite Marie Curie's house. He used to read my brother and I Lewis Carroll; play Mozart symphonies. All three were supposedly autistic ... It feels as if autism was always there in my past, unsuspected, unseen, but somehow part of the fabric of life.

One day, I Google Asperger syndrome. I suspect I may have a mild version of some of the symptoms, and, like all autism parents, have been asking the question: am I the reason? There is a vast amount of information, even online tests one can complete, with leading questions such as: *would you rather go to a library than a party?* Well, yes. But then I know plenty of people who would answer in the same way.

First, I read an article by a music critic who identifies as Asperger's. He says that, for him, conversation is like 'gas in the air', but when he listens to music he feels at home in the world. 'Intense, aggressive, claustrophobic rock'n'roll ... music that repeats a lot.' I feel the skin tighten on my face. I've always liked this sort of stuff. The Velvet Underground, Talk Talk, the German bands ... and the repetition of ska, dub, James Brown, John Lee Hooker ... I would much rather play a repeating pattern than improvise. For me, there is far more satisfaction – a physical, visceral pleasure, with only the pressure of one's fingers on the strings allowing any sort of tonal or timbral variation – in playing the same riff over and over again. It engenders a trance-like state, endorphins flow, anxiety levels drop. Is this what an autistic child feels when repetitively bashing a toy? Feeling 'at home in the world'?

He mentions 'thinking in pictures', the title of a book by an American professor of animal science, Dr Temple Grandin, who also happens to be autistic. I always 'see' music, too. If a fellow musician is teaching me a chord progression I can only retain it by rendering it visually, memorise it as a shape, a map of co-ordinates on the fretboard.

Then I find a blog by someone who defines herself as 'Aspie'. She lists a summary of her characteristics: *A profound need for solitary time and the deep fatigue that follows without it ... a wearyingly empathetic, emotional nature ... extreme sensitivity to light and sound ... desperate need for visual organisation, driven to distraction by clutter ... burn out rapidly from group socializing ... have to remind myself to make eye contact during conversation ... thinking in pictures ... ability to write, systemise, memorise information ... masking, adapting, blending in over the years.*

I'm going red. She's describing me. Or, at least, sometimes she is.

Am I 'Aspie'?

Is Asperger's the source of the anxiety I've felt all my life?

Most of her symptoms I have to some degree, especially the visual order. A sock poking out of a half-closed drawer menaces me, the hand-soap tap the wrong way round causes tension; the coat hangers all have to be facing the same way. But then I don't always need to do something about things being 'out of place'. The uncomfortable feelings pass.

The burnout from socialising in large groups I know well. Much later, I discover the excellent *The Electricity of Every*

Living Thing, by Katherine May, a writer with Asperger's, in which she describes habitually retreating to quiet rooms at social gatherings. I've always done this. At a recent house party, I found myself alone in an upstairs study, and thought: I'm here again. Sound and light, too. Hand-dryers, train door beeps, competing voices in pubs are all too loud. Skies and screens too bright. And the masking. I did a lot of masking (and drinking) in my twenties and thirties to survive social situations.

Something the blogger doesn't mention is collecting, a classic Asperger's trait. Perhaps it's a male thing. I think back to my obsessive boyhood interest in James Bond, the vast collection of memorabilia my brother and I amassed; the way I always needed to arrange the books and records in date order. Before that it had been fossils. All boys have their enthusiasms, but I wonder if I didn't take longer than him to grow out of ours.

Interestingly, she also writes that, when focusing on creating art, the world 'disappears'. When I wrote songs as a young man I could easily spend four or five hours shaping, sculpting, refining an idea, surfacing with surprise at the end of a long day. It always reminded me of playing as a child, the complete absorption in an activity.

Of course, these revelations may only be revelations for me. We can never be sure how others see us. I recall a friend once saying, 'Your knowledge of music is almost autistic.' But then he was misusing the term, in the same casual way people say, *oh, I think he or she might be on the spectrum.*

Perhaps I should do an online test. One day, maybe.

It's some consolation to learn that a great number of artists and musicians are thought to have the syndrome. In fact, I always suspected Nick Drake might have had Asperger's. Along with the old movies, it's his records that have been on repeat in my new, soulless Surbiton flat ...

One day in early summer I find myself in Chelsea. I take the King's Road onto Old Church Street, and keep walking past the walled gardens of fine houses. High up on a building set back from the road, I see a carved cow's head. Number 46a was once a 19th-century dairy, but in the late 1960s it contained a recording studio – Sound Techniques – and it was here Nick Drake recorded his peerless trilogy of albums. I've come on a pilgrimage.

Connoisseurs often remark that the records created at Sound Techniques have a uniquely rich, colourful sound. This was partly because of the first-class house engineer, John Wood; partly the equipment, much of which was homemade (and later sold to be installed in top US studios), and partly because of the odd shape of the room. There was a gentle gradient to the floor, a drainage requirement from the days when the cows were hosed down. An overhanging office dominated one side of the studio, and in the centre, a high ceiling had been created to provide a bright space in which to record strings. When the studio first opened, however, it was clear this renovation didn't provide the desired effect, so string players were moved to beneath the office, where the low roof gave a natural resonance – enabling a big sound from a small section. It was here, in 1969, that a 12-piece ensemble sat to record the discreet, Delius-influenced parts on Nick Drake's 'River Man'. He sat in the centre of the room, beneath the high ceiling, and, unbelievably, recorded his guitar and vocal at the same time as the string players.

I've been thinking a lot about Nick recently, reading the books about him as well as listening to the albums. Retro-diagnosis is a futile, perhaps even pernicious activity, but the more I read, the more I become convinced he had Asperger syndrome.

These are some of the known facts about his life. He taught himself in less than two years to become one of the most accomplished finger-style guitarists in the country, a feat that would have taken obsessively high levels of concentration. The figures in his songs are mostly repetitive, cyclical patterns (at Cambridge, contemporary and string arranger Robert Kirby described Drake's right hand as being 'like a machine'), deeply attractive structures for an autistic person. Similarly, his melodies and lyrics use much repetition, have the quality of incantation.

It's well known he was 'shy' and 'sensitive', a socially awkward individual who stuck to the peripheries of social events, as if always on the point of leaving, but these vague terms belie deeper problems. He had an intense need for privacy, was uncomfortable being touched or touching people; indeed, the world seemed so overwhelming for his too-open senses that a record company employee once remarked he was 'terrified of everything'. Most tellingly, perhaps, there seemed to be no anger or malice in his personality. People who knew Drake use the same phrases: 'child-like', 'innocent', 'unspoiled', 'not of this world'. Kirby said he was one of the few people he'd met who was completely pure and honest. (In *George and Sam*, Charlotte Moore lists this lack of guile as one of the blessings of her sons' autism. Many autistic people can neither tell nor detect a lie, due to their lack of a theory of mind. In fact, a neurotypical child's first lie is a major developmental milestone – when he or she first realises that another person doesn't know what they are thinking, and are therefore free to deceive them.)

Most of these autistic traits are of a piece with the role of seer-poet Nick Drake adopted. This is what people expect a romantic, lyrical troubadour to be like: fragile, remote, unknowable. It's possible that Drake, aware of his supreme difference, used his choice of career to mask the symptoms of ASD. If so, he might have been spared the exhausting struggle to maintain a facade of normality that people with Asperger's suffer. But in the songs, his turmoil is palpable. Many of his lyrics seem preoccupied with problems surrounding speech, anxiety at a perplexing failure to communicate with others. In 'Hazey Jane II' he declares that if songs were more like words in a conversation, everything would be fine. In 'At The Chime Of A City Clock' he admits he doesn't know what a face 'is for'. Moreover, for a singer-songwriter, there is a striking lack of metaphor or word-play in Drake's lyrics, relying instead on the use of naïve symbols, natural phenomena such as suns, moons, seas, rain, trees. He seemed unaware that the meaning they had for him might not be the meaning they had for others, that their significance might need to be translated somehow. He was baffled when his albums didn't sell.

The breakdown that followed Drake's commercial failure is more complicated. A withdrawal into silence took place. Stories exist of him sitting absorbed for hours, staring at his shoes or the sky, unwashed, nails grown out, not speaking. It seems undeniable he was suffering from depression at this point, but there could also have been an underlying autistic regression, common in people with Asperger's in their late teens and early twenties, where there is a loss of self-care, the ability to speak. Today, perhaps, Drake may have been given an Asperger's diagnosis from his psychiatrist, and not merely the prescription antidepressants which eventually killed him.

Idle speculation maybe, but if there had been more awareness of autism – virtually non-existent in the early 1970s – his life might have been saved. High-functioning autism has many co-occurring conditions, including depression, and the latest statistics from the National Autistic Society are that people with ASD, especially undiagnosed, are nine times more likely than members of the general public to commit suicide.

The carved cow's head is as far as I get on my pilgrimage. The studio closed in 1974. But it's been worth making to commune with the singer whose songs I've been playing daily.

Many years after Nick Drake recorded 'River Man' at Chelsea's Sound Techniques, I had my own small brush with the studio. Back in the early 00s, during set-breaks, I used to drink at the pub opposite the old dairy, The Pig's Ear – it was just around the corner from one of my venues. In all that time, around a decade – until I discovered the story of the studio by chance on the Internet – I wasn't aware that the building with the carved cow's head was where Nick Drake created 'River Man', in author Ian MacDonald's words, 'one of the sky-high classics of post-war English music', and one of the most important songs in my life.

25

Things Behind
The Sun

AND SO THE routine of travelling to Germany every
three weeks to see Emily begins. I buy a new wheeled case,
an ergonomic rucksack, a keep-cup for the countless coffees.
Surbiton to St Pancras; St Pancras to Brussels; Brussels to
Frankfurt; then a bus to the suburb. Twelve hours, if there are
no delays. Every aspect of the process becomes well-honed. I
carry separate change bags for the different currencies, wear
rubber soles for swift passage through customs; I know the
code for the vegetarian cafe's loo at Brussels station off by heart.
Sometimes it takes an immense effort to remember if I need to
find the Eurostar or the Deutsche Bahn train. But I'm always
looking forward to seeing Emily, singing to Emily.

On the first visit, during the long wait for a connection
at Brussels, I sit in the cafe, writing and watching the world.
Groups of teenage Interrailers pass by. They look the same as
they did when I was their age: Dylan caps, flip-flops, big bottles
of water. Festival wristbands, sunburn, shiny foreheads. Eating

burgers, or struggling with improvised luggage made from IKEA bags or laundry sacks. I feel warm towards them, their excited young faces, their body odour and hormones. I wonder if Emily will ever be part of a similar crowd.

Turning my gaze outwards, across a wide plaza, a group of young women in business suits, laughing and stumbling slightly, emerge from a bistro. Will Emily ever do this? The conjecture about missed futures is becoming tiresome, but I badly want her to fall out of a cafe at noon with her work friends one day, tipsy, sharing some scurrilous joke. I want her to enjoy those carefree moments of pleasure that the young take for granted.

When Anita opens the door to the apartment that evening, I'm convinced Emily will have forgotten me. But the corners of her mouth turn up, a smile appears, and her face comes alive with recognition. Happiness explodes in my chest. We run and chase each other down the wide corridor, roly-poly, bounce, tickle, cackle with laughter. I spin rings, throw footballs, play shakers. Every so often she stops, takes stock – appears to remember me all over again – and the smile that closes her eyes spreads across her face, causing a feeling of wellbeing to surge through me. She rushes up excitedly, as if she is about to give me a hug, but doesn't seem to know how to complete the action. At one point we clash foreheads, and I wait for the scream to come. But none does. She is unstoppable, a whirlwind.

I take down the guitar from the top of the wardrobe and play a song for her. 'Wish You Were Here'. She immediately falls under its spell. Her right hand makes a sign, a pinch grip with thumb and forefinger like an 'A-OK'; '*Ooh!*' she cries hoarsely, and throws her gaze to the floor in concentration. Her entire demeanour changes as I strum away. I sound good. Ironically, the apartment has better acoustics now all my stuff has gone.

Later, at the kitchen table, I talk with Anita about the progress of the autism therapies (slow-moving; Emily will start them soon), and the first day at kindergarten (end of August). The atmosphere between us seems to have improved somewhat. She admits she has dreams where our daughter can speak, too. I say that Emily's dream-voice is always wondrous, even when she's just swearing.

Anita sends me a look, unsure if I am joking or not.

'She's our little miracle,' I say.

We both have tears in our eyes.

And it is here Anita tells me the results from the genetics test arrived. No evidence of Rett's or Angelman syndrome was found. Dr Maier and Dr Schroeder at the children's hospital have now finally confirmed Emily's diagnosis as autism.

Time stands still for a second, seems to bend back on itself. Then relief hits like a wave.

So, in the end, the news didn't come with a flash of light, or any sense of ceremony. Just two estranged people sitting at a wooden table in a kitchen in Germany, talking; a few words the culmination of the pain and anguish of the last two years. Emily can now join the club, the great worldwide community of neurodiverse people who somehow all fit under the umbrella of autism.

Briefly, I wonder if we'll ever know whether the fragile site on chromosome 2q13 was the cause of her condition. In a sense, it doesn't matter. It's only parents who have a deep emotional need for answers. Emily is the same – herself – regardless.

I feel strangely optimistic. At last, we finally know where we are, and can move forward with ensuring Emily has all the help she needs for the journey ahead.

But back in Surbiton, the reality that I'll be seeing far less of my daughter begins to dawn. For the past two-and-a-half years she has been my constant companion, and now she's no longer with me.

I'm in tears most days. On the train into town one evening, I'm seen. A woman across the carriage, reading a *Metro*. I turn my face to the window, to hide my red, swollen eyes. But I know that train criers are compulsive viewing. I always stare. No matter how hard I try to look away, I'm inexorably drawn to them. What has happened? A redundancy? A break-up? A bereavement?

June becomes July. From my lounge window I watch high cumulus clouds drift over Long Ditton rec. I play my old vinyl records, looking out at the beckoning witch's fingers of the cedar trees in the park. Something about the recurring, waking dream – Emily and I at sea, shipwrecked, perhaps – sends me back to Kate Bush's *Hounds of Love*. Not side one, with its bright, upbeat hits – 'Cloudbusting', 'The Big Sky' – but the dark, conceptual suite of songs on side two, 'The Ninth Wave'. I now hear it – see it – through the lens of autism.

'The Ninth Wave' tells the story of a young girl lost at sea at night, following some unnamed disaster. As she drifts, waiting to be rescued, she slips between consciousness and nightmares. In Graeme Thomson's biography of Kate Bush, *Under the Ivy*, I discover that the idea for the song-cycle was inspired by a childhood dream of Kate's in which she found herself on a raft in the middle of an ocean, with no shoreline in sight. Yet she wasn't afraid, and certainly didn't want to be rescued.

'The Ninth Wave' is different. The girl is terrified by her situation. Listening with new ears, it strikes me as nothing less than an aural depiction of what severe autism might be like.

The centrepiece is a trio of songs, beginning with 'Under Ice', in which urgent cellos establish a sense of dread. Then, in 'Waking The Witch', voices of family members implore the girl to wake up, point things out, but go unheeded. Disembodied sounds of church bells fade in and vanish; a helicopter swoops overhead. A sudden, incomprehensible, staccato babbling strikes up, like the tape of a computerised voice cut up into hundreds of pieces, thrown into the air and reassembled at random. Behind this, deeper voices menace. Drums thunder, an unidentifiable instrument (a guitar? A keyboard?) wails; a shout from a megaphone warns the girl to *get out of the water*. The track is approaching a peak: sensory overload. Meltdown.

Then there is merciful release. 'Watching You Without Me' floats in on a steady, calming tempo, but something has happened: the girl has lost her ability to communicate. In the whispered backing vocals, hard to decipher, she tells us that *we can't hear her*, a line Thomson calls the album's 'saddest, most bereft' moment.

Eventually, she is rescued, although only in a metaphorical sense. In the deeply affecting 'The Morning Fog', she is brought back to dry land by the love of her family. A happy ending, of sorts.

Staring at the back sleeve and inner bag of *Hounds of Love*, I notice Kate Bush appears as the girl in 'The Ninth Wave', partially submerged in water, wearing a life jacket. She is also strewn with wild flowers – an allusion to John Everett Millais' famous painting of Ophelia in the river that hangs in the Tate. Bush had a special interest in the picture; she kept a modernist version, the *Hogsmill Ophelia*, in her home recording studio. A memory returns. Millais' *Ophelia* was painted in Ewell, near Surbiton, and one summer's day, back when Anita was pregnant with Emily, we took a walk there. Ewell, appropriately enough, is from the Old English *aewell* – the source of a river, or spring. I recall finding the exact spot on the bank, and looking up the flowers in a field guide I'd bought in a charity shop, intending one day to teach our daughter their names. *Dads should know stuff*, I kept telling myself. I was preparing to become a father. It's a hopeful, happy, innocent memory, one at odds with the darkness of 'The Ninth Wave'.

Another book – or rather, two books – reassure me the way I've always spoken to Emily, as if she understands, is correct. Naoki Higashida's *The Reason I Jump*, and its sequel, *Fall Down 7 Times Get Up 8*, are revelatory insider accounts of severe autism, written by a nonverbal Japanese boy using an alphabet grid – a qwerty keyboard drawn on cardboard. Both were translated into English by novelist David Mitchell and his Japanese wife, the writer KA Yoshida, themselves autism parents.

The Reason I Jump, written when Higashida was 13, consists of brief Q&A chapters that reveal an astonishing breadth of emotion. In an interview, Mitchell says the book confirmed his suspicions that autistic people feel what everyone else feels, they merely can't show it, hence the 'lack of empathy' myth. Indeed, he says that this fundamental mistake – confusing a cognitive impairment with a *communicative* one – could be this decade's 'big bad wrongness' about autism. As a result, Mitchell and Yoshida changed how they interacted with their autistic son, engaged with him more, and, crucially, expected more back. Their boy's understanding of situations improved, he self-harmed less, seemed happier. Of course, Mitchell adds, he couldn't be sure these changes wouldn't have happened anyway, but *The Reason I Jump* helped him to 'turn a corner'.

It has helped me turn a corner, too. I've always suspected Emily felt a lot, and perhaps had thoughts she couldn't express, always imagined there was more going on in her mind than she was able to show. And when I discovered that playing music for her unlocked her ability to interact, I saw flashes of potential I maybe wouldn't have otherwise detected. (It's a depressing fact, but human beings are hardwired to assume that if a person can't speak then they can't *think*. I admit I fell into this trap.) But *The Reason I Jump* confirmed there could be an articulate intelligence behind the silence.

This is not the same as saying there is a 'normal' child trapped inside an autistic one, as many anguished, misguided parents believe. Higashida merely offers plausible explanations for his behaviour, his stimming, or why he doesn't make eye contact.

In the second book, *Fall Down 7 Times Get Up 8*, Higashida is a young man in his early twenties. His eloquent – and, above all, concise – descriptions of what must be chaotic experiences are beautiful to read. Prose as clear as a Japanese mountain stream. But the subject matter is not always easy to stomach. He admits that wordlessness is 'agony', and that nonverbal autists are the loneliest people in the world. In addition, he says they are 'always listening'. Apart from the worry that Emily will suffer in a similar way (and I'm just hoping there was some post-teenage angst in Higashida's observations, although I doubt it), I will continue to believe that she, too, is always listening, and never speak 'over her' as if she isn't there, always as if she is.

Germany. Late July. I'm pushing the buggy towards the playground in the wood. It's a hot, sultry afternoon, and I'm singing George Harrison's 'Here Comes The Sun' for Emily. We stop at the swings. I sit her on my knees, place her small hands on the metal chains on either side of us, and once I'm sure she's gripping, up we go. Higher and higher, making the trees disappear for her, then reappear again. She makes contented coo-ing sounds, and I feel her body relax.

I let my mind wander to something that's been preoccupying me: planning her third birthday party, in late October. She will be over in England. Perhaps we could go to Long Ditton rec, visit the swings? It will be a homecoming …

When she tires of the motion, we walk along the path by the stream. Red admirals and cabbage whites flit about in the shade. She shows me she wants to push the buggy with both hands, so I let her. She walks ahead, a tiny Goliath.

'We're in *Germany*,' I say. 'Will you remember?'

The words I said to her as she stared at the ever-changing patterns of the stream, the first time we walked in these woods, and I tried to fathom what was in her mind. The thoughts of Mary Jane. We had only been in the country a matter of weeks. The phrase, and the question, somehow epitomises the hopeful tenor of that period.

I start singing another song.

Twinkle, twinkle, little star, how I wonder what you are …

Do I understand her slightly better now? I know she is sensitive, that she has an inner complexity I often catch glimpses of, but which she still has no means to express, except by a gesture or look, or a wordless sound.

On the way back to the apartment there is an unexpected explosion of vocalisms from her, attempts at speech. Strings of babble, loud and excited. Wild stabs at consonant-vowel combinations, like someone trying to play an instrument with no knowledge of a scale. But the will is there – I can hear it – to express herself verbally, with sound, with language. I copy her noises, turn them into words. Hoping, hoping.

At bedtime, after more songs, I read her *How to Hide a Lion*, one of the few age-appropriate books she responds to. She clambers up onto the sofa, smiling, giggling, eager to join me. Admittedly, after a few moments she loses interest, sprawls over the pages, tears at them with her fingers, dribbling. But she wanted to participate, join in. Be near others. I'm certain now that music increases her sociability. Then, when I see her yawning, I lift her up, singing the old favourite – the Beatles' 'Good Night' – and feel her body slump, ready for sleep.

She doesn't go off straight away. I listen from the lounge

as she laughs to herself, and makes odd sounds in her cot. At one point, she utters a long, incredible 'word', dozens of syllables long.

If only I could speak her language. If only I knew what was going on in her room – in her mind. It strikes me that Emily is in her room in two senses. Not only in her bedroom, but alone in her own mental world, just as Clara Claiborne Park's daughter was in her 'citadel'. She is happy there, for now; and beyond loved by Anita and I. But there is no growth in the citadel. It's our duty to coax Emily out of her room, to take her with us, so that she may grow, and find her place in the outside world.

I listen for a few more moments. Finally, there is silence.

Back in Surbiton, I have another dream in which Emily can talk. We are in a strange house with a cooker in the hall. A pot bubbles on the hob. Dream-Emily reaches up and puts her arms through the gas flame, hugging the scalding saucepan. She doesn't register any pain. Alarmed, I pick her up, put her over my shoulder, and walk down the corridor. Suddenly, she asks: 'Can I get down now, please?'

I'm amazed. She can speak! It's a holy sound, a voice from the mountain. We enter the lounge where family and friends are sitting in armchairs, drinking tea and eating huge slabs of carrot cake.

'Listen to this!' I announce. 'Emily, say it again.'

She struggles, like a stutterer, but manages to get the phrase out: 'Can I get down now, please?'

A wave of astonished excitement sweeps through the room, as if a talking alien had descended from a spacecraft. I allow Emily to slip gently to the floor. I'm in a state of rapture, leaping and dancing around. Soon we all are. She can *speak.*

But Emily can't stop: one childish observation or announcement follows another. Questions, demands, summaries. And this little girl's voice that is perfectly 'her', an extension or expression of her radiant personality – sunny, happy, laughing Emily – this little girl's voice that has never been heard before echoes around the room.

'Shall we go and bounce?' I ask, jubilantly.

Her face cracks into a huge smile.

'Yes, Daddy!' she says, and I put her on a trampoline that just happens to be in a corner of the lounge. Facing me, she raises her arms above her head and I take her hands.

'One, two, three, four – BOUNCE!' I say.

Soon her hair is leaping crazily as she jumps up and down, giggles becoming howls of laughter.

'Higher, Daddy, higher!' she cries.

'One, two, three, four – BOUNCE!'

I hold her under her arms and rocket her up as high as I can on the word 'bounce', her head almost touching the ceiling.

'Higher!'

'One, two, three, four – BOUNCE!'

'*Higher!*'

'One, two, three, four – BOUNCE!'

I wake up.

I'm alone, in my bedroom in Surbiton. The grey shapes of furniture stare back at me like a reproach. My phone glows on the bedside table. It's 4:50am. A milk train sounds in the distance, dragging its long ghost note. Cortisone burns in my stomach. The apprehension that what I've just experienced wasn't real – that I've been tricked, fooled, cheated – crushes me. I lie in the dark, shaking, gripped by a feeling of utter hopelessness. Emily can't speak, and will never speak.

26

Cloudbusting

A HOT SATURDAY in August, and I'm walking up the hill towards Alexandra Palace, north London. A great blue arch of sky stretches above, and around me immense distances are visible; the entire city laid out in the sunshine. I'm happy and excited, for I am about to see my daughter. Anita is over to meet a friend of hers, a surprise visit. I haven't seen Emily for three weeks, and I'm anxiously hoping she will remember me.

I arrive late at the meeting point. A text informs me they have already been to the play area and around the boating lake. So where are they? I make my way to the summit, and head for a wooded area to the right of the palace. The sun has brought out the crowds. I pass a disabled girl in a wheelchair. Her face is twisted into the headrest, as if pushed back by g-force, yet I see humour in her eyes. I know she is enjoying a day out, just like everyone else here, and that gives me comfort.

Eventually, I spy them on a path beneath a line of tall trees. Anita is standing next to the empty buggy, holding Emily on her shoulder. I walk over, my shirt damp, my heart galloping, but when I greet Emily she doesn't acknowledge me. No eye contact at all. I feel deeply wounded, and for a second, sure that we've lost the connection that has taken so much time to establish. But I know it is just her autism. The rush of stimuli in a busy, open space is occupying her to the full. She gazes stoically into the distance, squinting at the bright light. I notice she's wearing new, unfamiliar clothes: a red top with yellow elephants. Over this is a dribbler adorned by a picture of a bee, and the legend 'Bee Happy'.

I come close and whisper-sing a verse of The Emily Song in her ear. A faint smile rises to her lips. This is enough for me, and the great torment inside is soothed for a moment.

Emily seems hungry, so we make our way to a packed beer garden. I order a kid's portion of macaroni cheese and a Sprite for her, and we sit on a shade-less wooden bench in the midday heat. She's beginning to acknowledge me in small ways: as I feed her she claps her hand repetitively on my knee. I decant the Sprite into her water bottle. She can hold a drinking vessel with both hands now, a new development that I have missed in the weeks we've been apart.

Emily burps.

'It's her first ever fizzy drink,' Anita says.

Our daughter is becoming restless, wriggling, slipping off my knee. I decide to bring her over to the perimeter for a look at the view. We walk the short distance hand in hand, taking longer than anticipated – she's fascinated by her stretched, sharply defined shadow, keeps twisting around to stare at it.

Eventually, we reach the iron railings with their flaking coat of old blue paint, and I hoist her up on my shoulder. Colourful triangular flags strung above our heads snap in the strong breeze. I point to the Shard, Canary Wharf, the Post Office Tower, and beyond: the shimmering, dazed horizon. Cars flow by on the road below, and on the grass verge between our position and the tarmac there are abundant wild flowers. I name them for her, one by one (I knew that book would come in handy): ox-eye daisies, red campion, chamomile, foxglove, blue cornflowers, dandelions, buttercups, poppies …

The vista, the moving vehicles, the flags fluttering loudly overhead, the wind in her face all cause Emily to start stimming, excitedly flapping and twisting her hands. But she's smiling, laughing, making guttural sounds.

Happy.

Above us are bright, slow-moving clouds, separated by patches of deep blue sky. High summer. I think of Windmill Hill in Hitchin, flying kites as boy, Kate Bush and 'Cloudbusting'. I sing the song to her – shyly, as there are always people nearby – but I can feel her body relax, the soothing effect of the melody doing its work.

It's you and me, Daddy.

She stares straight ahead, the breeze ruffling her hair, silently absorbing the scene.

'We're on top of the world, Bear!' I say. 'If we had a Cloudbuster we could make it rain!'

When we've seen enough, we walk slowly back to the bench.

For some reason, a seated young couple are staring at us. Then I notice she's pregnant – he's stroking the bump beneath the table. They are thinking: one day we will do this with our baby, take her to look at the view on a fine summer's day. A simple, ordinary pleasure, costing nothing. *And you will*, I want to say as we pass them. The golden future that you picture will be yours, whether your child is autistic or not.

All too soon it's time for goodbyes. I give Emily a hug, and tell her I'll miss her, but she has already returned to her unreachable place. When they've gone, I head to the bar, order a pint of Moretti, and sit at the bench for a long time. I watch the numberless day trippers passing by in long lines. I don't know what to do with the absolute chaos of emotions I feel. Sadness and anger, elation and crushing depression, like some terrible drug comedown. I don't know when I'll see her again: there isn't another scheduled visit in the diary.

Oh, Emily.

Waitresses pass constantly with plates of wraps, fries, little wire mesh baskets brimming with chicken wings. It all seems meaningless. Was I just here with my daughter? Should I cut off contact, forget her? The thought shocks me. No, I could never do that. But sometimes the pain is too much. Sometimes I fear I am becoming a peripheral figure in her life. A ghost.

Shut up. You need a kick up the behind. You should enjoy what you've got. So many others don't have this. You should just enjoy the miracle that is Emily, whenever and wherever you can. *Bee Happy*.

After half an hour, I make my way to a bus stop on the road. I look up, and in the place where I stood with Emily, there is a different father and daughter. He's showing her the perfect white sphere of a dandelion seed head. She blows on it, and the delicate filaments disperse into the air.

I turn and stare at the grounds of the palace below. Joggers, couples, kite-fliers, families. The big sky above. Then I look back, and see that a woman has joined the dad and the dandelion girl, completing them.

*

Two days later, Anita sends a photograph from Germany. Emily has her back to the camera, and is wearing a small, pink, orange and yellow rucksack, emblazoned with a rabbit and a cartoon bear. It's slightly too large for her narrow shoulders. The caption on the text reads: 'First day at kindergarten soon'. I think of the children by the roundabout, on the way back from the hospital that day, their rucksacks in a heap. *Everywhere, futures are closing for her.* And at a stroke, that awful memory is erased, replaced by a feeling of boundless joy.

*

Each night, I trawl YouTube for videos about autism. I find an alarming documentary featuring interviews with older autism parents. They attempt to explain how the condition feels for their grown-up children: 'It's like being in a foreign country with an incomprehensible language.'

Some of the words they use haunt me. 'Outcast'.

I don't want my daughter to be an outcast.

They say that their kids are adults in all but name, and most exist in assisted living conditions, watched day and night lest they bolt and run into a road, or drown themselves in a river. Some can't even shower without help.

I feel, for a second, as if I'm going mad. Is this what awaits Emily? The thought threatens to overwhelm me, until I can't breathe.

I force myself to continue watching.

'People don't like folk they can't understand,' they say, 'it scares them … Society is comfortable accommodating people with physical disabilities – it sort of gets that now – but not learning disabilities.'

The common thread for all is 'the black hole of fear' when the safety net of education times out. There are very few support options past 21. The adult years are like 'falling off a cliff', one mother says. 'The cliff', it turns out, is autism parlance for this watershed, when the choices for low-functioning autistic individuals are either living at home or in state-funded residential care. They talk darkly about the abuse that is allowed to happen in these places. But it's inevitable, the parents say, that our children will eventually end up being looked after by strangers, when we are no longer alive.

One couple, who care for their autistic son at home, are asked what their plan for the future is. They reply:

'Don't die.'

*

It strikes me that autistic characters in film and television are nearly always high-functioning, whereas severe, nonverbal autism is practically invisible. I read in the *Guardian* that 'autism is very much "in", part of the international conversation about identity in a way it's never been before', but is that all autism, or only one type? There needs to be a new *Rain Man*, I decide. A four-Oscar picture, not about an autistic savant, but a regular, nonverbal autistic person coping with daily life.

I re-watch *Rain Man*. The main character's autism is surprisingly well portrayed. Dustin Hoffman, as Raymond Babbitt, is transfixed by the shadow of a moving car, engrossed in a tumble dryer spinning; melts down when a smoke alarm goes off. He rocks from foot to foot, copies phrases – echolalia – and rarely makes eye contact. I had expected to find an emphasis on Raymond's savant skills, but, interestingly, they are not central to the film. His extraordinary facility with numbers isn't a plot motor; he doesn't mastermind a bank heist or avert an asteroid strike with it. Yes, there's the casino scene where his brother, yuppie on-the-make Charlie Babbitt, played by Tom Cruise, uses Raymond's calculations to win back the money he lost on a bad car deal, but nothing pivotal. Yet it's what everyone remembers from the film, the 'special skill'. In an interview, David Mitchell says the general public seem to have a deep-seated need for this gift, and adds that he's tired of people asking him what his son's 'superpower' is. Charlotte Moore, in *George and Sam*, says the need arises because the skill 'validates' their autism. It hardly surprises me though; as an identical twin, I'm used to being asked if my brother and I are telepathic. The answer is: no, don't be ridiculous.

By the end of the movie, in the Hollywood manner, Tom Cruise becomes a better person, and enlists to look after his brother, while all Hoffman can do is crack a single joke – he has no character arc. It's an odd, muted little film in which not much happens. Yet it was a four-Oscar blockbuster. Why? Because of the sensitive portrayal of the relationship between the two characters. Raymond Babbitt's humanity – revealed by Hoffman's nuanced, sympathetic performance – and Tom Cruise's ultimate recognition of it, was hugely important for the film's success, precipitating a new era of autism awareness.

I watch *Rain Man* three times in a row. On the third viewing, I notice Raymond *does* have a character arc. It's shown in the final act, when the brothers, in an office, lean into each other and touch heads. Unusually, Raymond leads. This gesture – symbolic of the gulf between the neurodiverse and neurotypical brain – is the only time Raymond initiates physical contact with another person, his version of a hug. (Earlier, Tom Cruise's attempt to embrace his brother prompts a meltdown. Cruise becomes aggrieved. 'Hey man, I was just trying to give you a hug.') It's at this moment that tears come. I realise Emily has never hugged me. Once or twice, when she moves closer after I pull open the Velcro clasp on the hand tambourine, or when she runs grinning towards me down the apartment's long corridor, arms wide, I think it might happen. But it never does. I suppose I'll just have to accept she's not a 'huggy' person.

27

Song To The Siren

GERMANY. THE END of August. Emily's first day at pre-school arrives. I leave my Airbnb at 7:00am, cross the *autobahn* bridge without stopping for once, and take a hidden wooded path that runs beside a drained, disused swimming pond. Slugs glisten on the muddy crater, a black cat lopes in the elderflower; the air is damp and heavy with earth odours. I walk on, through a graffiti-d underpass and head down a long, straight boulevard of silver birch. The sun is rising on my left, just cresting the treetops. I'm excited about the day ahead. I hope the unfamiliar setting and the many social negotiations won't be too much for Emily.

When I push through the door to the apartment, I see her with the pink, orange and yellow rucksack on her back, the one from the photograph. I'm overwhelmed with pride. Her first day! After brushing her teeth, I follow her and Anita to the car, watching her stumbling, shambolic gait, this small person clinging to her mother's hand. Barely containable emotions are just below the surface. Everything means too much. I need to be careful.

When we arrive at the kindergarten it's deserted, besides two of the key workers. They show us upstairs, and, after a brief exchange, Anita leaves for work. Emily and I are on our own.

Things swiftly unravel.

Within minutes, the room is packed with parents and their charges. I must shake hands, smile; remember names. I don't understand their questions, as they're all in German. Soon it is I who is exhausted by the social negotiations. Then it's Emily's turn. She begins to have crying jags – meltdowns – as the bombardment of sensory information becomes more and more overwhelming. I take her away from the commotion, clap hands, sing; whisper encouragement, anything to calm her.

The two key workers, Luisa – young, voluble, Spanish – and Clara – fortyish, quiet, German – don't speak English. (Or rather, *I* don't speak German.) Actually, that's not quite true. They have minimal English, just enough to make communication possible. But there's always one word that derails the conversation.

'What does Emily like for breakfast?' asks Luisa.

'Porridge,' I reply.

A blank look.

'*Wie bitte?* Sorry?

What is the German word? You know it.

A silence grows.

Come on. Try to think.

A rictus smile from Luisa.

Try harder. *What is it?*

Finally, it comes …

'*Hafer.*'

'*Ah, Haferbrei!*'

'*Ja, Haferbrei.*'

Gloomily, I reflect that language is everything – the username and password to life rolled into one. 'The master-tool of speech' as Clara Claiborne Park calls it in *The Siege*. And its deficit is the handicap that Emily will have to overcome each day she is alive.

Presently, we are asked to go downstairs for breakfast. I sit with Emily at the low table, surrounded by her new playmates and the key workers. I explain in a mixture of English and broken German: no plates or knives near her, please – she'll just sweep them onto the floor.

A candle is lit, and Emily follows the puff of smoke as it rises slowly to the ceiling. The twining, uncoiling, bluish-white rope causes her to start waving her hands – stimming – and, shockingly, Luisa copies her.

'*Fliegen, Emily, fliegen!*' She says, smiling. Fly, Emily, fly!

The other children join in. She encourages them. Soon everyone is flapping their hands as if they are birds.

This is all a mistake. I'm convinced now. She should be in a special needs nursery, not an *Integrativ*. Her contemporaries are so far ahead, almost a different species. They eat their bread, lift their cups steadily to their mouths, ask questions and point to things. I'm stricken with fear. How on earth will Emily navigate any of this?

'You're doing just great, darling,' I whisper in her ear, and I mean it. But then tears instantly fill my eyes and I have to avert my face.

This is where she must learn the survival skills necessary for the outside world. We've kept her insulated for too long, and now it has to be faced: real life starts here, today, and she's not ready yet.

After breakfast, in the cramped cloakroom, Emily has meltdown after meltdown. Parents and children are squeezing past, the mums and dads hanging up their kids' coats, the boys and girls changing into their *Hausschuhe*. Searching for Emily's shoes, the contents of her rucksack spill across the floor. Snacks, hairclips, tissues, spare socks, water bottle, nappies. The other little ones are jumping up and down in front of me, tugging at my sleeve, asking wide-eyed questions in incomprehensible German. A clamorous, overpowering crossfire of social interactions. Emily screams and cries. I bring her to the door to cool her down. Walk her. Hold her. *Sing to her.*

Should I take her home?

No. We've got to get through it.

The first activity is free play. On a mat, there are Lego trains and spaceships, built last term by the older children. Emily strides in, squats down, and begins systematically dismantling the models, throwing each piece over her shoulder as she goes. I quickly intervene. It might have been funny if I hadn't caught the appalled looks of other parents. She's being 'disruptive', yes, but the word implies malicious intent. I must remember that Emily's behaviour is entirely appropriate to her condition, her autism.

Clara suggests we move to another room. We find ourselves in a high-windowed gymnasium. There are still boisterous children running everywhere, but Emily's mood seems to improve. We play chase; I help her jump up and down on the crash mat. I realise I'm slyly demonstrating to Clara how I interact with my daughter. Every so often Emily stops what she is doing and smiles, distracted by something she's seen outside: a small plume of white smoke exiting a chimney, against the blue August sky. She studies it with painterly absorption, considering the compelling, ever-replenishing shape. I stop and do the same. The form is constantly changing yet somehow oddly static. I notice how this contradiction – repetitive motion and reliable stasis – is having a calming effect on her.

We're recalled to the playroom. Song Time. Children and parents sit in a circle on little red cushions. Emily is chaotic, a ball of unpredictable energies, and I need to restrain her as she perches on my knees. She lunges into the boy next to me, accidentally putting her hand in his crotch. I apologise to the startled child and worried mother. But then the song, and the clapping, become too loud – *Guten Mor-gen! Guten Mor-gen!* – and Emily is in tears again, howling. I ask if we can sing a bit quieter, please. Generously, there is agreement.

Emily calms, and introductions are made, going around the circle, one by one. As our turn approaches I tense as I wonder what I'm going to say. And in which language. Should I mention her autism?

Here it comes.

I'm on.

I begin with my customary disclaimer, '*Ich spreche nur ein wenig Deutsch*' – I only speak a little German. Then: 'I'm James, and this is my daughter, Emily.'

Several parents smile and nod.

Next, I summon all my courage, and smiling as brightly as I can, say: 'She's autistic. *Autistisch.*'

There is silence around the circle.

A wave of discomfort sweeps the mums and dads in the group. Some lower their eyes, others turn their faces away. A few seem fine with it. Luisa regards me with kindness.

'You don't have to say that.'

'It's not a bad thing,' I reply, still smiling to demonstrate that I am 100 per cent proud of my daughter.

The introductions move on, and my neck and back prickle with relief. They need to know that this is not 'a naughty girl'.

There's a Down's syndrome child in the group, and I find myself wishing that Emily had some dysmorphia, too, that her behaviour could be 'explained'. But autism is the invisible disability. It doesn't come with a wheelchair or a white stick.

Half an hour later, outside by the sandpit while the children play, I speak to the Down's syndrome girl's mother. It seems we have much in common. She's seeking a one-to-one helper at the nursery for her daughter, Mia. I make a mental note to find an assistant for Emily. I'm introduced to Mia. Her beautiful, doleful Down's eyes acknowledge me. She extends a small hand, waves. Then looks away, with a bashful grin.

'Hello, Mia,' I say, 'that's a lovely smile you've got.'

Just at that moment, sad-eyed Clara appears at my side, suggests I take a break while she walks with Emily. I agree, reluctantly, and watch as she leads my daughter away. For the next 20 minutes, I'm anxiously thinking of excuses to join them. I catch glimpses of Emily, hand in hand with Clara, or alone at the top of the slide in her pink cardigan, squinting into the strong sunlight.

I must let her go, out into life.

Eventually, Clara walks slowly over with Emily, and suggests we should go home. But why? I ask. We've been here for less than three hours, she's not upset. But Clara is adamant: it's for the best. I accept the judgement, but I'm not pleased.

I change Emily's shoes, gather her belongings, squeeze everything into her rucksack, all the while gripping her with one hand. She won't sit still for a second, slipping off the low wooden bench in the cloakroom as if it was coated in butter. Then I clip her into the buggy, open the wooden gate, and we're out, charging for the bus. Emily is in her strange, subdued mood – as she always was after nursery in Surbiton – seemingly processing all that has just taken place.

Back in the flat, after some lunch, Emily is relaxed, contented, throwing toys around on the floor in the lounge. I sit on the sofa and sing the Beatles' 'Mother Nature's Son' for her, changing the 'son' to 'girl'. She grins, clambers up and sits beside me. And there we remain for a while, content in each other's company as I sing my a cappella repertoire. 'Let It Be', which brings a smile. 'Bridge Over Troubled Water', 'The Long And Winding Road'. Finally, when I intone Time For A Nap, another made-up song, the melody plagiarised yet again from 'Three Blind Mice' (I owe the writers thousands), she leads me to her cot.

Later, when Anita returns from work, we talk about the morning. Why, I ask, was Emily so calm when we got back to the apartment? Was she relieved to be out of the kindergarten, or had the social maelstrom stimulated her in some positive way? Was she, I wondered, proud of how she had eventually steered through her first, difficult day at pre-school? As always, it's conjecture: she has no means to tell us.

I mention my discomfort at the stimming incident, the children copying Emily, led by Luisa. *Fliegen, Emily, Fliegen!* Anita insists it was a teacher's method, a way of normalising 'bizarre' behaviour for the others. Now I think of it, Luisa wasn't mocking her, but smiling genuinely. The children, too. What's more, Anita says, Clara sending Emily home when she was happy, and not melting down, was another technique. Quit while you're winning, as the saying goes. They know what they're doing, I just have to relax; trust them.

Back at the Airbnb, exhausted, I go over the day in my mind. I was like an amateur dad at certain points, a novice – flustered, close to losing control when I couldn't find Emily's *Hausschuhe*, and the contents of her rucksack scattered across the floor; parents and kids stepping over me, Emily howling. I was out of my depth. A helpless state of near panic in the face of escalating noise and chaos, Emily twisting out of my grip, ready to run heedlessly into the kitchen to pull out knives, wires; knock over brooms. This, I realise, is how Emily might have felt during her meltdowns, only much worse.

I put together some *Brötchen*, Gouda and cherry tomatoes, cover them in *Kräutersalz*, and pour a large glass of red. Then I fire up my laptop, and find the video for This Mortal Coil's 'Song To The Siren' on YouTube. The clip, which has over four million views (quite a few of which are surely mine), begins. Autumn leaves turn, a monochrome Elizabeth Fraser appears, her hands clasped demurely before her. She opens her mouth … and that sound comes out. The emotions that I've kept in check all day swiftly rise to the surface.

I cry and cry and cry. I can't seem to stop. The music – its spaces, those wintry silences – somehow evoke Emily and my feelings for her. Her autism. The rucksack. Her future.

Oh, Emily.

Wave after wave of racking sobs come, my body shaking, heaving; more like a bout of dysentery than a crying fit. An evacuation.

What are we going to do?

I gulp air into my lungs, my face a mask of tears and mucus.

When the attack finally recedes, with the last notes of the song, my breathing under control, I feel cleansed: washed through with better chemicals. I go to the bathroom. My red, distended face stares back at me in the mirror. I look as if I've been beaten up. I allow myself a small, dry laugh.

I think back to the morning, Emily with her rucksack on her first day. Why is the image so powerful for me? Yes, it probably is sentimental, 'cute', a little girl wearing a slightly too-big-for-her backpack. But there is something else: it embodies hope. The rucksack is a symbol of a purposeful, integrated working and social life. It is an emblem of the tool kit she will need for her future. The rucksack will go through many incarnations. It will change to a satchel, a briefcase, a student tote bag, then back to a rucksack again, on the 7:30 to Waterloo …

Hope dies last.

28

The Rainbow II

I'M BACK IN England after four days in Germany. Emily has been at the kindergarten for over a month now, and after that fraught first day, has settled in well. The key workers say she 'brings so much to the nursery', and she now has a one-to-one assistant, a German teenager, who 'fell in love' with Emily when she saw her, apparently. For the time being, my fears are assuaged.

Emily is making progress at home, too. After weeks of hard work from Anita and the kindergarten staff, she can now just about hold a spoon without dropping it, and with great effort, scoop up a little porridge, and bring it falteringly to her lips. She's mastered the most basic skill for life on earth: feeding oneself. Although a trivial accomplishment for other children her age, this is a huge learning milestone for her. There is no failure in autism …

But, I realise, with a selfish flicker of regret, if she can use the spoon herself, and not be fed by others, she must sit squarely facing the table in her high chair, with the bowl in front of her. The days of her feet resting on my knees are over. She's growing up.

One day, in the apartment, I witness another breakthrough. Anita demonstrates. Standing in the long corridor, she hands Emily her door keys. Emily walks to the locked front door, tries to open it from the inside. I watch in disbelief. Now, beyond any doubt, I'm certain there's cognition she can't show us. This is a child who doesn't respond to 'stop' or 'no', let alone her name, and yet she appears to understand the concept of a lock and a key.

September becomes October. The preparations for Emily's third birthday visit to England preoccupy me. I must have the small table in the kitchen ready for her, at the right height. I must go to Kingston to look for a travel cot. I must buy decorations, a card, toys, wrapping paper. I've already bought her main present, an iPad: an investment for the next five to ten years. She can't use it now, of course; it would go flying across the room. But maybe if the tablet was Gaffa-taped down somehow…? She could play with Brian Eno's 'Bloom' music App. At the touch of a finger a distant note sounds, and a visual, like the ripple from a pebble thrown into a stream spreads across the screen. Touch again: another note-chime and ripple. Soon the screen is filled with circles that bloom out and overlap, and ever-repeating, colliding tones, forming strange harmonies and dissonances. You're creating your own ambient piece.

I've staged Emily's birthday over and over again in my mind:

the presents in the morning, lunch with family – my mother and her partner Ian are visiting from Yorkshire – then cake, and afterwards we could head over to Long Ditton rec, see if Emily would like to go on the swings … I know it won't be precisely like this, but it's become, through dress rehearsal after dress rehearsal, some sort of mystical culmination for me.

The last Friday in October. Anita and Emily arrive in the afternoon on a Germanwings flight from Frankfurt. Our daughter is three years old tomorrow.

For a late lunch, we go to the Italian restaurant opposite Surbiton station, like we used to in the old days. It's deeply strange, sitting in this place with the project of a shared future cancelled, although I detect an odd harmony between Anita and I. Our only project now is Emily.

We talk about the ABA therapy that she will be starting next month in Germany. The autism centre in Frankfurt finally got in touch with a schedule. I mention the unit at the local school that our old neighbour Anna told me about, still privately hoping we can co-parent here some day …

Emily sits in a high chair and we take turns to feed her a child's portion of *Pasta al pomodoro*. Soon it is everywhere, on her face, her hair, her clothes. She smiles, and twists in her seat, making unpredictable sounds that I find I'm unusually anxious about. But I can see she's enjoying the experience, a meal out. Then we head back to my flat, and I still haven't got used to calling it that.

On the way, I buy a last raft of toys from a charity shop. Coloured sensory balls, a small tambourine, a plastic turtle, a fluffy elephant. It's a slowly darkening October day. There are leaves underfoot, pumpkins in Poundland.

When we return, I begin putting up decorations and balloons in the lounge. I can hear Anita in the kitchen telling Emily it's her third birthday tomorrow.

'*Deine Geburtstag … Ein, zwei, drei Jahre!*'

Then the three of us play chase, charging through the small rooms. Emily squeals and hoots with joy. 'From The Morning', the last song on Nick Drake's third album, *Pink Moon*, is playing; the lines about endless summer days reliably bringing back my earliest memory: crawling, aged three, on the new grey carpet with its new-carpet smell, light flooding through the panels of the front door, in the hall of my childhood home in Hitchin.

At 5pm, with the afternoon slipping away, I prepare Emily for a walk. I put on her striped rainbow hat, zip up her padded blue anorak, and we step outside. The air is cool, autumnal. I point out the V formations of Surbiton geese flying high above, heading for warmer climes. I don't mind that she doesn't follow my finger.

We make our way to Long Ditton rec, following the path by the railway cutting. Without warning, a train hurtles past over our heads. A smear of red, yellow and blue. I'm expecting Emily to jump, but she stands transfixed, smiling. We listen to the tons of metal crashing through space, a sound like the roar of a huge crowd, and inside this funnel of noise, the strange ghost tone: a choir singing in unison. This is what seems to hold her attention. Of course. I remember reading that some autistic children hear musical notes as 'friends'. The enormous, sustained tone is her Big Friendly Giant.

We walk on. My phone beeps. A text from Anita saying she feels quite emotional, now that Emily is almost three. I put the handset back in my pocket, but it goes again. Another communication, but this one makes me stop and stand motionless on the path. Attached are two photographs of Emily in profile. In the first, she's a day old, still in hospital, the bruise from the forceps showing above her right eye. The second is a shot from earlier today, the same profile.

'Our beautiful girl,' reads the message.

We continue past the steel railings, under the chestnut trees and the beckoning witch's fingers of the cedars, crunching dead leaves and conkers underfoot. We pass the benches painted boot-polish brown, the small grey marble fountain, then take a left at the cricket pavilion, and head for a central spot near the swings and the slide. The sun is sinking behind the tree line. Long, moon-landing shadows extend from the goal posts on the playing field. This is the park where those odd words came to me, seemingly a lifetime ago. *You can have a bit of everything, my darling. Think of life as a feast – you can have a bit of everything.* I had no inkling of what was to come.

I say the words out loud now, as dogs run and jump nearby, and a father and son kick a football.

'We're here again, but we're both older!' I say. 'You're *three* tomorrow!'

I don't know if she understands, but I tell her anyway. 'That's – what?' I attempt a quick mental arithmetic. Maths was never my strong suit. 'Over a thousand days!'

I wish her thousands more.

Another train sounds in the distance, in G, I think.

Emily runs around in a circle, holding my hand; slips, pulls herself up, then begins running again. The last rays are gleaming on the high bar of the swings. A strange, glowing cast of light is enveloping us. The cedars stretch in benediction now. She stops, and stares into the setting sun, squinting with that singular expression of hers. Her calm, sentient gaze: taking in the world.

A memory returns, from the holiday in Gran Canaria, the first time I really noticed the expression. It was the day before her first birthday. We were at a seafront restaurant late one afternoon, Anita, Emily and I, Andrew, Carrie and little Billy. It had been raining; we were undercover, with our buggies and toys and wet wipes and mess. Much wine and beer had been drunk; aioli shrimp consumed. Emily was crying as usual, but the rain had cleared so I decided to take her for a walk. I planted her onto my left forearm and we made our way around the tables to the nearby sands. It was that melancholy hour, when people pack up their towels and beach bags. The tide was far out, the sky a white screen of cloud. I realised in that moment it was only the second time she'd seen the ocean.

'This is the sea, Bear!' I said to her, bobbing her tiny body up and down. Her crying had stopped, and I noticed her expression, that circumspect squint. She was looking at something in the distance. And there, above the horizon, I saw it, too: a rainbow. But not like the one glimpsed from above on the mountain road a few days earlier, astonishingly circular, this was a faint fragment, a fading shard, gradually being erased by the cloud cover.

'Look, Em, another rainbow!' I said, stupidly, as it was

she who had noticed it first. I remembered wanting to show her 'all the beauty in the world'. She didn't need my help. We stood and stared, the two of us on the deserted shore, until it was gone.

I didn't know Emily was autistic then, but she was, and that thought brings consolation now, back in the park, watching the sun setting over the swings. She wasn't stolen from Anita and I, wasn't an alien or a changeling, she was herself, her autistic self, all along.

Emily.

I crouch down beside her on the path, and offer up a prayer to a God I don't believe in.

Dear God, when Anita and I are dead and gone, whoever is looking after Emily – please don't let them hurt her.

Then I pull her close.

'Do you remember?' I ask, something I say to her a lot. 'Do you remember when we saw the rainbow?'

Her silence prevails, the little girl who cannot speak, her detached, stoic expression, staring into the heart of light. The most extraordinary person I have ever met. And there, in the park, with the sun going down, casting goal posts and benches and leaping dogs in gold, my foolish heart breaking, I speak softly in her ear:

Our beautiful girl – may you always see the rainbow.

And the child who has never once spoken a word in all her thousand days, turns and whispers in my ear the meaning of life.

EPILOGUE

Wealth

Surbiton, October 2019

OF COURSE, SHE never whispered the meaning of life to me in Long Ditton rec, Surbiton, the day before her third birthday – she'd already given me that many months before, without words. Not the meaning of life, exactly, more how to live. Be in the moment, in touch with the natural world. Like the Buddha, free from material desires. Like Mark Hollis in his self-imposed silence. Like Nick Drake, or William Blake, able to perceive heaven in a wild flower. But much more, be your best self. Adopt the autistic lack of malice and guile. Be tolerant; celebrate differences. Be kind.

Emily's third birthday came and went, exactly as I'd imagined it, almost. (I'd dressed her that morning in her finest party frock. It wasn't until lunchtime that Anita pointed out it was the wrong way round.) After a few days, she returned to Germany with her mother. In the weeks that followed, I waited, hoping that a text would arrive announcing she had spoken her first word. But one never did. We were about to enter the Time of No Reply.

*

'Be your child's anthropologist,' said Donna Williams, the writer and ASD consultant who was herself autistic, when asked on a television documentary what advice she would give to autism parents. With this in mind, I return to Dorita S. Berger's superb book, *Music Therapy, Sensory Integration and the Autistic Child*. Reading it makes me feel as if I know Emily better, that I understand her mechanism slightly more, have an idea, at last, of 'what is going on in that noodle' of hers, on a physiological level at least.

Here, as they say, comes the science bit.

Berger, a concert pianist and trained music therapist, begins by reminding us that one of the main causes of erratic behaviours in ASD is the autistic brain's difficulty in decoding and integrating the profusion of sensory information in the world. These behaviours – the stims, such as hand flapping, rocking, jumping, humming, etc. – may seem 'weird' to neurotypical humans living happily on planet earth, but to the neurodivergent person they come naturally, seem normal. As their systems perceive it, they are living on an alien planet, and stimming is merely an adaptive response to incoming sensory information that is confusing and often painful. The behaviours are *normal* for that system. We must remember, she writes, that it is us who speaks the foreign language we think they should adapt to. They see neurotypicals as the aliens, not the other way round. With this humbling reversal in mind, she then submits that music creates a 'safe space', restores order to chaos, brings sensory balance and a feeling of wellbeing to the autistic brain. So how does something as abstract as music bring this about?

All sensory information is first processed by the lower, 'old brain' (500 million years old, known as the *paleoencephalon*). How we respond to external stimuli – sound, light, heat and everything else – depends on this ancient gatekeeper. The incoming information is sieved to assess whether it is 'safe'. If deemed to be unsafe, the system goes into upheaval: fight-or-flight mode. Nothing will reach the higher, cognitive, neo-cortex ('new brain') until the danger and fear issues have been resolved.

To the autistic system, a majority of sensory stimuli appear to be threatening. For whatever reasons (a deficit of neurones in the cerebellum is one theory), it seems unable to register sensory information properly and respond appropriately. Thus, tactile, auditory and visual inputs are perceived as discomforts, eliciting fear responses: those calming behaviours, the stims. And very little can be learned when the cognitive, intellectual, new brain can't be engaged – the old brain is simply too busy, stuck in fight-or-flight mode. Precisely how physiotherapist Jane described Emily's Low Sensory Threshold, back when Emily was one.

It explains much of Emily's other behaviour, too. Faced with this sensory overload, a bombardment of more information than it knows how to deal with, in no recognisable sequence, with no 'rhyme or reason', the autistic brain simply ignores it. Hence her lack of response to language, pointing, people, pictures, calls. Her brain was – is – under perpetual siege.

Upheaval. Bombardment. Siege. Fear. Words like these make me marvel at Emily's courage, how tough she is, how resilient. To go through life coping with that much adversity, and, moreover, do it with a smile and a laugh. *Emily the Lionheart*, indeed. This is what she has really taught me. This is how to live – with courage, and a sense of humour.

But back to the theory. Unknowns and surprises cause anxiety, confusion, tension, and, ultimately, meltdown. Ritualistic behaviours provide comfort, 'sameness' – repetition of something that is known, dependable. Music provides a similar function: a quieting factor that causes the old brain to calm down. Crucially, music doesn't need to be 'interpreted', it merely provides an environment: the safe space. (Or, to quote another Berger – John – from his essay collection *Confabulations*: a song constructs 'a shelter from the flow of linear time'.)

When I sang 'Row Your Boat' to Emily during her crying fits, many of which I now know were meltdowns, I was doing what all parents do instinctively with a distressed child. I don't claim any great insight for that. What I didn't know was that I was providing a safety blanket for her scattered system, her permanent, innate condition: autism. Furthermore, during 'Wish You Were Here', when I noticed that Emily was 'present' as long as the music played, I wasn't aware that the brain, treating auditory information as a means to assess the environment, automatically hones in to rhythm and linked sound sequences. The brain 'tracks' a piece of music, and stays tuned in for its duration.

This is how music creates the safe space that allows learning to happen, how it reduces the autistic system's physical stress so the brain is able to process information calmly. All music (even the most inaccessible piece of *musique concrète*) contains repetition, patterns. The brain loves patterns, but the autistic brain *really* loves them, seizing upon order in chaos. The brain 'snaps to attention' when exposed to a repetitive rhythm. Moreover, music is a sedative, causing relaxants such as dopamine to be released, thus reducing the fight-or-flight response. With music playing, a threatening new situation becomes more acceptable to the old brain.

Once this safe environment is established, music therapy then aims to bring about a certain level of functional sensory adaptation, urging the sub-cortical, instinctive, old brain to adopt new standards of how it assesses threat. Nothing less than a re-wiring of brain circuitry, *conditioning*. (And we shouldn't be worried about this word. All learning is conditioning: riding a bicycle is instructing the old brain how to deal with balance and gravity under new circumstances.) Of course, this all depends on the individual. It could take a lifetime for any adaptations to occur.

And here I have to admit to a problem with the terminology. 'Music therapy'. I wish it had a different name. It sounds slightly trivial, as if it might have more to do with entertainment than treatment. But in fact all the arts have their established practices, and music therapy works just like the more serious-sounding occupational therapy, and all other allied therapies – conditioning of the old brain by the new brain. Teaching an old dog new tricks, as the cliché has it. Yes, music is enjoyable, 'enriching', but in this context that is not its central function. As Berger points out, cherry-flavoured medicine is still medicine.

For people with ASD, music is not a leisure option or a luxury, but a crucial learning tool for life.

More and more of Emily's behaviour is elucidated. The three basic, old brain sensory systems, vestibular (balance and gravity), proprioceptive (where the body and limbs are in space) and tactile (touch), work together with the higher visual and auditory systems, enabling the brain to make sense of the world.

In an autistic child these systems are dysfunctional. A vestibular system that doesn't work properly leads to clumsy, wobbling movements (I think of Emily running), and a stim called 'toe-walking' – the brain attempting to stabilise the body by walking on tiptoes. Another stabiliser is the physical act of jumping, and is why occupational therapy uses a lot of trampoline. Music therapy can work in tandem with OT, using synchronised instrumental and verbal pulses along with the jumping ('One, two, three, four – BOUNCE!' was my instinctive version of this). This helps to internalise rhythm, leading to better-organised body movements, motor control, eye focus; the brain 'forgetting' for a moment what it can't do, and allowing adaptations to occur.

A dysfunctional tactile system can also be adapted using music. Emily enjoys being held and tickled, but has some tactile defensiveness: a hug feels slightly threatening for her; she pushes you away. However, it only *seems* like a hostile advance because the brain is misinterpreting the feeling. Introduce music, which the brain 'attends' to, captured by the constant rhythm and melody, and it sees the hug as safe, leading to the release of dopamine, and less physical inhibition. Moreover, sound vibrations from the instrument playing in the room are enveloping, sending a tactile message that is soothing, acceptable. (Which is perhaps why Emily places the palm of her hand on the guitar as I play, to get nearer to the safe place.)

As Berger expands her theories, she goes on to offer a possible explanation of nonverbal autism, of precisely why Emily has no words.

The auditory system of an autistic person is using 'survival' or 'ambient' hearing – experiencing all sounds at once. Overload occurs, leading to the brain not knowing what should be discarded or kept, never focusing on a particular sound for long enough. (I think back to the first psychologist's meeting, asking about the phonemes, those distinct units of sound that a child, listening for speech patterns, builds language from, and whether Emily was being confused by having two native languages. She wasn't. She was unable to latch onto *any* phonemes.) Add to this an unusual sensitivity to certain frequencies (*hyperacusis*), causing the middle-ear reflex that shuts down intake of loud sounds – the ear's version of a squint – and there is a direct impact on attention span, and thus the acquisition of receptive and expressive language.

And this is why music therapy can be one of the most useful interventions for a nonverbal autistic child – the use of phonemes as part of a song can be one of the best ways of learning them. (Good old '*Knives, forks, spoons*', The Dishwasher Song.) This is because, unlike the visual arts – a painting, for example – a song unfolds, evolves over a period of real time. The brain *awaits* its note-by-note formation, tunes into each sound until a unified whole is revealed. The brain 'listens' to music (as opposed to merely passively 'hearing' it), searching for specific information.

Can music ever be perceived as an *unsafe* space for an autistic child? Very occasionally, playing a tune on guitar to Emily, she becomes agitated, and bursts into tears. I stop immediately and change the song (early on, I quickly learned that she's not a great fan of Country & Western), but it makes me think certain sound elements of a particular piece might be painful for her. (It could, of course, have just been my rendition.)

Berger confirms this suspicion with a story about a nonverbal autistic boy who was brought to her for music therapy. His parents told her he responded to sound oddly – became agitated in a crowded shopping mall, yet didn't flinch at a loud car horn, but was always calm when a television programme had musical content. During their first session, when Berger began playing the piano and singing accompaniment, the boy became distraught, 'satelliting' about the room, crouching in corners, sometimes screaming with his hands over his ears. She instantly moved to softer sounds, recorders, etc., but over the following weeks nothing really seemed to work. Then, one day, he noticed a large gong on the instrument rack and slammed it hard with a mallet. As the incredibly loud, almost unbearable sound reverberated around the room, the boy stood still, smiled, and started to laugh.

This account immediately makes me think of Emily and the train as it hurtled above our heads in Long Ditton rec; my surprise when she didn't jump. The infinite range of frequencies of a piano, from several hundred piano strings – possibly out of tune; it later transpired the boy had perfect pitch – plus a singing voice, reflecting, bouncing off the studio walls seemed like an intolerable tsunami of sound to him, an assault. With his ambient, survival hearing, he was experiencing all tones at once, leading to sensory overload. Meltdown. Madness. Hell. The gong, on the other hand, although enormously loud in comparison, was a *single* sound with hardly any overtones. Like the train's huge note, it was his Big Friendly Giant.

This is why a music therapist, in the initial assessment, is careful to ascertain which instruments are tolerable to the individual. (I realise it was a stroke of pure luck that Emily found the guitar and voice combination acceptable, otherwise I would have packed the instrument back in its case, and we would never have found our unique connection.) Indeed, the therapist must have no assumptions that music is always 'fun', or that the patient needs closeness or connection, or even that they are perceiving harmonic, rhythmic and melodic content as such.

And this begs a crucial question. What does a nonverbal autistic child like Emily hear when listening to music as opposed to speech?

How a person makes sense of sound patterns depends on how they sequentially track them. Music is a repetitive looping of sounds, whereas speech is all stops and starts. Emily recognises a tune – the 'A-OK' hand gesture, her gaze thrown down to the floor, the hoarse '*Ooh!*' when 'Wish You Were Here' begins – which is enormously encouraging: her auditory tracking must be good. To remember a piece of music is an incredibly complex feat for the brain, depending on the retention of a series of melodic notes in the short-term memory, and their later reconstruction in exactly the same order. Speech, on the other hand, seems harder for Emily to track. The challenge, Berger says, is to transfer this music tracking ability to the speech tracking centres of the brain; adding that most of the nonverbal children she works with eventually form word sounds.

Often, linear auditory tracking may be *too* good in an autistic child, resulting, as mentioned earlier, in perfect pitch. She writes of another nonverbal boy who screamed when she sang a song in a different key to the one in which she originally presented it. Pitches heard once are recalled 'exactly as memorised'. And here I wonder if Emily recognised 'Shall we go and bounce?' as a *musical* phrase, not language, and somehow linked it to the physical act of jumping up and down. I always say it 'in the same key', as it were, *sotto voce*, conspiratorially – musically – in my lower register: *Shall we go and bounce?* What if I said it in a different key, would she still take my hand and drag me to the makeshift trampoline? I haven't been brave enough to try yet, in case that precious piece of communication is lost.

Berger conjectures that it is unlikely music exists entirely for pleasure. Given the brain's efficiency, its evolution towards ever-more economic use of incoming information, would it create something irrelevant to its survival? No, it would seem much more likely that the brain 'invented' music to help us adapt to our surroundings, reduce tension, and express emotion.

And this leads to a question I'm often asked when people

learn that I play music for my daughter, that it remains our main form of communication: is music a language?

In many ways music is the opposite of language. To begin with, they are processed in two different parts of the brain. Music, unlike language, doesn't challenge the neo-cortex to interpret information or provide meaning, it's understood instinctively, intuitively by the old brain. (Helped no doubt by the ancestral relationship: *before language there was music.*) Language is trickier. A nonverbal autistic person's tracking system codes language – with its unpredictable rhythms and high frequencies – in a non-sequential way, possibly rendering it completely meaningless. *Why are you constantly making that strange sound?* Music, on the other hand, can be tracked as it is – a song is accepted as a 'sound event' that makes sense.

Throughout this book, I've been using the vague term 'music' when in fact I should be qualifying it as 'live music'. Emily reacts to recorded music – the radio, or a CD (Bach's *Passion*, floating from the mezzanine in Surbiton; the Beatles 'Love You To' in the kitchen in Germany), but the difference when music is played live is marked. This may be due to the fact that recorded music is 'compressed' (flattened) in a studio, and the brain tunes out continuous, predictable stimuli, but also, because of her survival hearing she lacks an auditory figure ground. ('Figure ground' – a term borrowed from photography – refers to what is heard in the foreground, with non-essential sounds tuned out to the background.) To someone who hears all sounds at once, as equal, a single live instrument such as a guitar or unaccompanied voice provides a strong focus.

Berger also explains why Emily turns her face away from the sound when listening to music. A neurotypical brain, on hearing a sound, instinctively needs to *see* its source, the two senses 'confirming' each other. But the overloaded autistic brain needs to *shut down* one sense (usually visual) in order to process another. What seems like inattentiveness – a child not looking or listening – is actually the opposite. Naoki Higashida says he doesn't make eye contact when you speak to him because he is '*looking* at' your voice (my italics), i.e. desperately trying to tune into, code, sequence and recall the information contained in what is being said. Once again, a behaviour that seems abnormal or 'antisocial' is completely normal for that person's system. (Think of what happens, after the initial instinct to link sound and source, when we try to concentrate on something complex. When we ask a passer-by on the street for directions, say, and they proceed to give a lengthy, verbose explanation, or when we listen to a Mozart symphony on headphones, what do we do? Close our eyes.)

In the final part of her book, Berger breaks music down into some of its basic elements – rhythm, melody, dynamics, form – investigating the impact of each on the autistic child. Rhythm is the brain and body's organiser (it's also a social unifier – drums are found in all cultures). She writes about a third nonverbal boy she worked with who moved chaotically and was distant, unreachable. When she played a pulse on a drum she saw that it completely 'reorganised' him. He stopped moving, walked towards the sound, his once erratic paces becoming synchronised to the beat. The story reminds me of Emily's response when I drummed along to Neu!'s 'E-Musik'. The 'switch' that occurred: alternating current to direct current. This is known as *entrainment* – the body's internal rhythm aligning to an imposed, external beat, a direct result of the auditory cortex being located close to the motor cortex.

Within rhythm – strict time-keeping – there can be patterning, or accents. Eighth notes, 16th notes, triplets. Playing around with a rhythm as a drummer does. Berger observes that her nonverbal patients become more attentive, and imitate more word sounds when there is patterning. (I think, slightly smugly, of how I did this instinctively in The Emily Song. '*Em –i – ly, cha, cha, cha,*' – three quick handclaps, a triplet.)

In Berger's section on melody, Emily's response to the 'funny' lick in 'Wish You Were Here' is illuminated. She observes that quick, short, staccato melodies induce laughter, which is important for encouraging social behaviour in autistic children. Laughter, one of the earliest human calls, is always cohesive for a social group. When I play the lick, Emily laughs, which makes me laugh, too, and I play it again for her. A chain of communication is set in motion.

The dynamics of a piece of music, loud to soft, soft to loud – diminuendos and crescendos – can also be a social unifier. Emily and I do both love a trash-can ending …

But perhaps the most important element for an autistic child, from a learning perspective, is *form*. Music has form, shape – like a story it has a beginning, middle, and an end, and harnessing this can be a unique way of developing attention span. 'Attention', as Berger points out, is actually just 'anticipation'. A piece of music's form makes the brain attend, wait in a state of anticipation, staying 'on-task' until it ends.

Music, then, could be the ultimate therapy, super-food for the autistic brain and body. It might be the single most powerful, and *direct*, catalyst in reorganising the autistic child's scrambled system. Music has the advantage of being a multisensory intervention, reaching all the systems – vestibular, proprioceptive, tactile, auditory and visual – at the same time, engendering development in organised movement, balance, sociability, motivation to learn, attention span, and, crucially, language.

Berger is careful to say, however, that music shouldn't replace other interventions, such as OT and ABA, but work *with* them. She is also careful to say that her findings are anecdotal, that these are just theories she's developed over the years with her colleagues.

So maybe this wasn't the science bit, after all. But when I finally come to the end of Berger's book, I'm convinced any autism parent reading it would be knocking over tables and chairs to enlist music therapy for their child.

*

'Would Dad like to bond with Baby?' asks the nurse.

Hell, yes.

I take off my T-shirt and hold her tiny, blanketed weight against my bare chest, one hand cupping her head, the other under her bum. I'm sitting in the same burgundy vinyl NHS armchair I was in seven hours ago, but the world has utterly changed. My newborn daughter is so hungry she's trying to eat her thumb, the blanket – me.

She is ten minutes old.

Within seconds, we are alone. Our brilliant team of doctors, nurses and midwives have left for other deliveries, which seems disloyal somehow. Emily – for that is what we've chosen to name her – is looking up at me with huge, frightened, famished eyes. The white, antiseptic room seems suddenly enormous. The only sounds are the buzzing of the strip lights and the muffled, far-off screams of labouring women.

Who's in charge here?

I am.

At this point in my life it's the longest I've been alone with a baby, let alone with sole responsibility for one. She is bringing up a greenish-black liquid, the meconium. With a start of fear, I realise I must distract her. No silence, not even a second, or she will start crying. So I sing a song, 'Blackbird' by the Beatles. It seems as if we calm each other in some odd way. I try some more – tune after tune; half-remembered words, approximate melodies. And in the breaks I whisper to her. *Darling, you did it! You made it. I want you to meet everyone, see your new home. There's so much stuff to see and do. We're going to have so much fun. It's going to be all right.*

Everything will be all right.

The night is massive and cold and black behind the high windows, but in our room, my daughter and I are safe and warm.

The memory of her first room returns quite often. Number 26, the maternity wing of a Surrey hospital. Sometimes, I try to picture all the rooms Emily will find herself in during her lifetime. Some of them scare me.

Rooms are existential. The great American novelist James Salter said life is meals, but it is also rooms. Often, I remember minute details of a room from the past, but not what took place there. Other times I remember *everything* that took place. Rooms are all about identity. When a child with a sibling is finally granted their own room, it's a major milestone on their journey to creating a separate self. I was ten when I left the bunk beds I shared with my twin brother for a tiny bedroom at the front of the house, and remember it as a turning point. *A room of my own*. I was virtually a grown-up. Rooms are *personal*. (And rooms have personalities, too, as we have seen with Sound Techniques, and Wessex's cavernous studio one.) They can offer solace and peace. In his song, 'In My Room', the Beach Boys' Brian Wilson saw his teenage bedroom as a refuge from a confusing, hostile world. He was, as he admits in another song, just not made for these times. Or perhaps he should have sung the times were not made for him …

Wilson is yet another musician who is supposed to be autistic. Surely, it would be more surprising if he wasn't. As Hans Asperger wrote, to succeed in the arts (or sciences), it helps to have a dash of autism. The online lists of eminent people said to have had the condition are long. Leonardo da Vinci, Michelangelo, Einstein, Newton, Darwin, Lewis Carroll, Emily Dickinson, W.B. Yeats, James Joyce, Wittgenstein, Bobby Fischer, Stanley Kubrick, Andy Warhol, Alan Turing, Bill Gates, Steve Jobs … And those are just the scientists, artists and writers. The musicians and composers are thought to include Mozart, Beethoven, Bruckner, Mahler, Bartók, Glenn Gould, James Taylor, David Byrne (yes, David Byrne who wrote 'Once In A Lifetime') ... Consider almost any artist and it might be possible to place them on the spectrum. Richey Edwards of Manic Street Preachers? Nicknamed 'Android' by his bandmates, a slightly 'flat' effect in person: Asperger's (as a recent biography, *Withdrawn Traces*, suggests). Bach? No one has put forward the theory that he had ASD, but when I listen to the *Goldberg Variations*, played by Glenn Gould, the music's architecture, its harmonic perfection, its mathematical rigour, seems to me to have an overwhelmingly autistic aspect. In fact, autism might even *explain* the classical composers. Think of that Mozart symphony again. It's unlikely a neurotypical mind could have created something so complex; that worked on so many different levels at once. Like the Silicon Valley hackers who are able to hold hundreds of lines of code as visual images in their minds, Mozart was someone who could see the many parts in relation to the whole.

Retro-diagnosing someone with a neurological condition many years after their death is a dubious practice, as already mentioned in an earlier chapter. But it's interesting how much of our civilisation and culture has been created or influenced by autistic adults. There is a slogan that runs we'd still be living in caves if it wasn't for autism. Indeed, the ultra-connected world we live in today – computers, the Internet, AI – are all courtesy of a man with ASD: Alan Turing. And now it seems the earth might even be saved from ecological disaster by a teenager with Asperger's, Greta Thunberg.

If the genetic code is deciphered one day, and autistic people, with their child-like absorption and ability to see details others miss, to 'think outside the box', are screened from humanity, then the world will be a poorer, more dangerous place. As the ancient scholar in *Wings of Desire* says, when mankind loses its childhood, it loses its storyteller.

*

Step back to the Time of No Reply, the weeks and months following Emily's third birthday. The phrase is the title of an early Nick Drake song, one that always came to mind when contemplating Emily's lack of speech. In a sense, Anita and I had always been in a time of no reply with our daughter, but the words of the psychologist (*Some children at age three say a whole sentence when before they couldn't say a word*), and Clara Claiborne Park, who writes in *The Siege* that she always had 'the number five' in the back of her mind, made me hopeful that this is when speech would come: between the ages of three and five. But it never did. At the time of writing, Emily – almost five – has yet to speak a single recognisable word.

Other skills have flourished, however. Around the time she started toe-walking – at three-and-a-half – she learned how to climb into her high chair, place her hands on the bib in an effort to fasten it, put her plate in the sink when she'd finished eating. Later on, she was able to locate the correct kitchen drawer for her bowl, close the *kühlschrank* after her mother had taken out the milk, and recognise (i.e. go wild with anticipation) the word 'Babybel'. She also developed some basic self-care skills: hoisting up her trousers or tights a notch while being dressed, pulling up the zip on her padded outdoor jacket. These actions were not elective or instinctive. Following a prompt, there was always a pause of a few seconds, where she would look away, then realise what she was meant to do, and do it. Yet these seemingly trivial advances are huge cognitive and motor leaps for her, a result of continuous, tireless intervention from Anita, and the team of ABA therapists who visit the apartment every week.

ABA – Applied Behaviour Analysis – is still a controversial therapy, 50 years after it was devised by the Norwegian-American psychologist Ivar Lovaas. Its goal is to encourage behaviours that are helpful to the child, and decrease those that negatively impact learning, or are harmful. This is achieved by the use of conditioning 'reinforcers', a treat when a task is successfully completed, a sweet, for example (Emily prefers blueberries). But back in the 1970s, 'aversives' – physical punishments – were also used, when an activity failed, or a behaviour persisted. ABA was popular with parents desperate to eliminate autistic traits such as stimming from their children, so that they may appear 'normal' in society – and it is this that is at the root of its unpopularity with the neurodiversity movement today.

ABA is a lengthy process, the 'analysis' referring to the detailed logging of every facet of the child's behaviour over many years. But the benefits can be immediate, affecting multiple aspects of their everyday life. An early breakthrough for Emily was transitions. Like a first-time novelist, she couldn't do them – each time we came back from a walk or the shops there would be a mini meltdown as we went through the front door. Then another when I opened the apartment door. But when I slipped her a reinforcing blueberry, an action that she found intolerable (going into a new situation) became associated with pleasure, and thus acceptable.

Behaviour that is 'harmful' or antisocial is more problematic. Between the ages of three and four, Emily began to self-harm, hitting herself in the face with the back or the palm of her hand at times of high frustration or meltdown. Distressing to observe for a parent, and worse for her, it thankfully became rarer the more ABA she received, and as she learned to exercise more self-control herself. The same with hair-pulling – adults and children – and the dribbling. She still bites occasionally, though, herself and others, something that will have to be monitored in the future.

*

Life for an autism parent is a never-ending learning process. My epiphany after reading *In a Different Key* – that I must celebrate Emily's condition – should have been the part of the story where trite lessons were learned and everything from then on was fine. But I soon found my conversion to neurodiversity was merely the first stage of a long undertaking. In his introduction to *George and Sam*, autism parent Nick Hornby says the process of acceptance can take years. Henry Normal, in his excellent memoir *A Normal Family*, says that he was unable to write about his autistic son for almost two decades, and is still 'a work in progress' in regards to his acceptance of him as such.

I have the occasional bad day, if I am honest, when I find myself imagining what a non-autistic Emily would be like, and then am immediately consumed by guilt and shame. If Emily didn't have autism then she wouldn't be Emily, and I wouldn't want that at all.

Here are a couple of things I have learned.

When I think back to those terrible, panic-filled days and nights, where the pressure to set therapies in place immediately was overwhelming – the clock ticking – I have a measure of distance. Early intervention is vital, but autism seems to be a condition in which brain maturity evolves over a lifetime. In Oliver Sacks's documentary *Rage for Order*, Clara Claiborne's Park's daughter, Jessy, is shown discovering a sense of embarrassment at the age of 37. The 'learning machinery' appears to be switched on long after the supposed cut-off point, the age of three, or thereabouts.

'The genetic syndromes are too scary to contemplate,' I said in the car, after the long series of tests in Dr Schroeder's office. I didn't know then that Emily's form of autism, classic nonverbal (or 'severe', 'low-functioning'; I prefer 'profound') would be easily as 'scary' as Angelman syndrome; her life chances just as limited. There will almost certainly be no job interviews, no dates, no marriage. I will never walk her down the aisle, or hold a grandchild in my arms. So why don't I feel the same terror as I did when I said those words? Mostly, it is because she is happy, which was the goal at the end of the long list of things I wanted for my daughter, four years ago. She has been spared, or is overcoming, many of the sensory issues (she gladly wears a black, punk-ish, mohair jumper – many an autist's worst nightmare), has no epilepsy (touch wood), only mild self-harm, and none of the dietary issues that plague children with autism. Happiness, that most elusive condition, is hers, for now. The only thing remaining on my wish list is for her to reach her full potential, whatever that may be.

Since reading *In a Different Key*, the neuro-tribal conflicts, fought largely on social media, have descended into an ugly exchange of accusations and insults. Extremists in the neurodiversity camp are lobbying for ASD to be removed from the DSM, the Diagnostic and Statistical Manual of Mental Disorders, which, opponents furiously claim, would lead to a disaster for autism research. The anti-neurodiversity faction insists that ND ignores low-functioning autism; that the condition is being taken over by those who see it merely as an edgy identity label. The problem seems to be that people on both sides can only see autism in binary, black and white terms. To celebrate or mourn? A 'blessing', or a curse? A medical condition or just a difference? I don't have a problem with accepting autism as a paradox, an unsolvable enigma. Emily is extravagantly, perhaps catastrophically, disabled. But she is also an affectionate, sensitive, expressive, delightful human being – with many as yet-to-be-seen capabilities – who just happens to experience the world differently.

She is both her abilities and her disabilities.

David Mitchell, in his introduction to *Fall Down 7 Times Get Up 8*, wrote that he hoped the book would dispel myths and misconceptions about autism, and, ultimately, promote the cause of neurodiversity. Awareness was his mantra, and it is mine, too. I shan't rest until people stop carelessly saying, *Oh, I think he-or-she might be on the spectrum*; until people stop assuming all autists lack empathy and are maths savants; until 'stimming' and 'neurodiversity' cease to have the red wavy underline in a Word document. And until people stop talking about a cure. Autism is not a disease, it's not an illness caused by a known biological agent; it's an innate, inborn *condition*. There is no cure.

But a drive towards another, darker form of autism awareness has recently come to prominence, in the UK, at least. The slashing of funds for special needs provision has led to a deep crisis in adult social care. At the same time, the shocking abuse of autistic and learning disabled people in Assessment and Treatment Units (ATUs) and certain care homes – institutions in all but name – has led to an outcry, and vital, urgent questions. What value do people with autism and learning disabilities have in our society? What does it say about us when such human rights scandals are allowed to take place?

I worry about Emily's future every day. The rise of the far right, especially in Germany, and the 'othering' of sections of the population – people of colour, people with disabilities; the LGBT, Muslim, and Jewish communities – is deeply concerning. What is ironic, and horrifying, is that although Emily is receiving the finest medical care today in liberal, democratic Germany, 80 years ago she would have been euthanised as someone with a 'mental deficiency'. Another of Hitler's 'useless eaters'. The Nazis, with their revulsion for 'weaklings' first practised their methods on disabled people. If the lessons of history are allowed to be forgotten, a catastrophe for people with autism and their families would certainly follow.

*

One day, during my first year back in Surbiton, I summoned the courage to return to the old house. I took the river path towards Kingston, crossed Claremont Road, then walked up Church Passage, past the lamp post where I used to pause on my midnight journeys home from work – noting that the crumbling wall had been repaired, the ivy cut back – and watched as the spire of St Mark's loomed into view. My heart was racing. I turned left at the end of the alley, walked a few more paces, and stood in front of the building with the Victorian fanlight above the front door, staring up at what used to be Emily's bedroom. Incredibly, the same orange curtains were still hanging. I tried to recall moments from my old life there, in the James Bond flat, the excitement and exhaustion of those early days with a new baby. The morning it snowed at 5:00am and we held her up to the window to look at the blue street below. The moment in the lounge when she took her first steps. The barbecues in the tangled back garden with the other NCT children. They would be starting in Year One, doing maths and English tests. Only Emily was on a different path.

Allowing the memories to come, it felt for one vertiginous moment as if none of it ever happened. Then I noticed something odd about the line of sight between myself and the house. I realised the great copper beech that Emily loved was no longer there. I turned and walked slowly away, through Church Passage, back to my new life on the other side of town.

Later that year, one chilly, misted evening in December, I paid a visit to my father and his partner, Joan, at their house in Kent. For various reasons, I hadn't seen them since they came over to Surbiton for lunch three years previously, although I'd updated them about Emily in the meantime. We sat in their living room, eating delicious lamb, green beans, and new potatoes, talking about my daughter, and Joan's intellectually disabled son. Richard was then 51, still in residential care, incontinent, wheelchair-bound, with difficulties swallowing. The staff liked him, she said, because he smiled a lot and was generally happy. She told me more about his childhood, how he was obsessed with locks and keys, weather reports; how he responded to music: Haydn's 'Tick Tock' symphony, No.101, being a favourite. I suggested he may be autistic. Joan said, yes, he could be.

There were moments of black humour – a story about a meeting at the care home, where the manager insisted Richard was making progress with dressing himself. Richard was sitting in the room with his underpants on his head. Joan and her then husband couldn't stop laughing. But mostly the stories were bleak. The time when Richard was rejected from a Steiner school ('we can't do anything for him') and they drove back from the appointment in tears. The time when Richard's epilepsy started without warning, aged eight, causing him to stop sleeping at night. Joan was hospitalised with exhaustion within a month.

At the end of the night, the last wine in the glasses, she reached across the table, placed her hand on mine, and I recalled the words that caused a shockwave of denial in me three years earlier. *I know the worry you're going through, my darling.* This time, her eyes were damp, and so were mine.

*

The following year, not long after Anita and I were divorced, I signed a book deal for the memoir about nineties music I'd been working on. When it was published, I left the gigs behind, and found other ways to earn money that still allowed me to write. The only music I play now is for Emily.

The present day. Emily is almost five. I still travel to Germany every few weeks. I take over the childcare for two days, do some work in the nursery garden, then return to England, with my pictures and memories of her. And each time I alight at St Pancras, I'm greeted by Tracey Emin's red neon light sculpture: *I want my time with you.*

Sometimes, when I walk through the door to the apartment in Germany, Emily looks straight through me, and it feels like a dagger to my heart. I hoist her up on my arm so she can smell me, sing The Emily Song so she can hear me, let her see me move so she can remember my actions. Other times she shrieks in recognition. I'm not sure if she knows I'm her father, or just the guitar man, here again to entertain her. But her smile: head thrown back, eyes tightly shut – a Stevie Wonder grin – torches up an Olympic flame in me. And I notice that, each time I visit, her autism is becoming ever more 'glaring', while, paradoxically, she is learning new skills. *She is both her abilities and her disabilities.*

The dream of bringing her up in the UK remains, for the time being, just that. While I'm in Surbiton, I only see her via WhatsApp or Skype, a happy little girl splashing in the bath, slick as a seal, or running excitedly through the apartment, flapping her hands loosely at the wrist, as if she wanted to throw them away. I have an array of musical boxes, shakers and, of course, a guitar next to me on the sofa, at the ready. When she hears one of these, she starts clapping, smiling, and if I'm lucky looks into the camera, and we make eye contact. I know from experience that without these props no connection is made. Sometimes, when these brief sessions are over, I'm on a high; other times, I feel as if I've lost her, and I exhale a long breath, and sit motionless on the sofa for a long time.

While I'm in Germany, music is still our main form of communication, our favourite thing. If she sees the guitar in the lounge, she becomes overwhelmed with excitement – throws her arms open, '*Ah!*' as if greeting an old friend – and drags the instrument hungrily over for me. Lately, with the help of ABA, and a birdsong book that emits calls with the press of a finger, she has learned that point-touching gets her something she wants (oh, the look of pleasure on her face), especially the guitar. This is not an instinctive neurotypical point, but still a clear demonstration of choice. An extension of this is sign language. Emily now has a basic gesture, the first and second finger of her right hand prodding the palm of her left, to indicate that she'd like to jump on a new mini trampoline, or be spun in a special revolving chair.

We also play a game that, although seemingly simple, relies on a series of complex cognitive feats from her. I throw a sensory football to a far corner of the lounge and she runs off to retrieve it. 'Give to Daddy,' I repeat, until she picks it up. Then she returns, secret smiling, delighted with this activity and its immutable rules; stands completely still, staring at the floor, and after a long pause places the ball carefully in my hands. '*Yay!*' I say, applauding, and give her the lightest of hugs, remembering she doesn't really like them.

My repertoire of songs has increased, along with Emily's array of responses. She now always 'sings' along (tuneless wailing, but still attempts at word sounds), and on the acoustic intro to Led Zeppelin's 'Over The Hills And Far Away' we do a sort of dance around each other, a reel, which she initiates. I've got 'Jealous Guy' down (the irony of singing the line about trying to catch your eye to an autistic child always makes me smile), and 'Cinnamon Girl', 'Moon River', 'All Apologies', 'Rebel Rebel', Zeppelin's 'Ten Years Gone' (instrumental only – are you kidding?) I do Pete Townshend leaps; spin on my heel like James Dean Bradfield of Manic Street Preachers; race down the corridor playing the guitar above my head like Eddie Van Halen on an ego, showmanship which delights her. Then I need a lie-down. In these breaks she perches on the trampoline, next to a window in the lounge, and considers the people on the cobbled street below. Sometimes I rise and join her. I study her profile, her long, iron-filing-grey lashes, her delicate retroussé nose, her fair hair held back in a single mauve clip on the top of her head.

She's a lioness. A tiny dancer.

She's a rainbow.

My late gift.

She touches the cold glass of the window; then her lips, and her fingers make the old shapes. I study her hands, so like my own, the camber of the third and fourth fingers. There is something self-contained, complete, in her familiar mannerisms, her singular body language.

I still wonder if she has a memory. Most of the time, I believe she does. An emotional or procedural memory, not one encoded with language. We are storied animals, but I'm convinced now that she remembers feelings, in the way a preverbal child remembers un-storied experience. Her concealed cognition –

the mysterious river of consciousness just below the surface that rises but rarely breaks through as expression – may always be her secret to keep.

Here, as we look at the street together in our rest from the music, she often tries to form a word, variations on a root. 'Breer' or 'bear'. Sometimes it sounds like 'beer'.

That's my girl.

Maybe there is a single recognisable word, after all.

How hard it is to stop this account becoming the success story everyone so badly wants, suggests Clara Claiborne Park in *The Siege*. All disability stories tend to move from darkness to light, but this one, hopefully, moves only from darkness to some kind of lucidity. There are no Disney happy endings with autism.

One morning, during my most recent visit to Germany – Anita at work, Emily at kindergarten – I find myself standing in our daughter's light-filled room, aware of the breeze and sounds from the street coming through the open window; the *crêpe suzette* smells of sugar and lemon that evoke childhood memories of Paris, and pause awhile. The lion print is still above her cot, which always houses her trusty white rabbit, but other things have changed. The space is cleaner. It doesn't resemble a child's room anymore, all toys are tided away – ABA rules, so she doesn't become distracted, stays on task. This is good: I won't accidentally tread on a musical bear and wake her up as I'm backing quietly out of the room after putting her down to sleep. The buggy, which she is too big for now, is folded up down in the *Keller*. The dummy that would usually be found in the cot is long gone; the changing table has vanished – all nappy changes are now to be carried out in the bathroom. The mountain that is toilet training is up ahead, yet to be climbed.

Emily is growing up fast.

There is a new white wardrobe in one corner. I open it, releasing a clean, woody IKEA smell, and one of freshly laundered clothes. I stare at them hanging or folded in neat rows, the array of colourful tops, trousers, dresses, skirts, all slightly larger than last year's. The hair clips and bobbles kept neatly in small boxes. Yes, Anita is a good mother.

Perhaps there is hope for the future, foolish hope, but hope nonetheless. I hope that when others see Emily's smile, her profound innocence, her strange dignity – her true colours – they will accept her, too. I realise that while she is in her room she is in autistic space, she is just herself. It's only outside that she may be judged. I straighten her sleeping bag, place the white rabbit beside it; fold her peach pyjamas, lay them over the rail of the cot, and close the door softly behind me.

One last picture of Emily. It's a month after her fourth birthday. We're in the back of a cab – a smart, clean BMW – on the way to the kindergarten. I'm in the rear passenger seat, Emily next to me on a child's *sitzplatz*. The driver is a young Muslim guy with a skullcap who smiled when he saw Emily, and helped her into the car, gently placing the seatbelt under her arms. Now, outside the smeared windows, grey, rainy Frankfurt is flashing by. We shoot over an intersection, and accelerate up a steep hill, overtaking bicycles and buses. Emily, although tired, is happy and excited to be in this novel form of transport. She twists and turns, eager to see the strange new rooftops fly past overhead. She's making noises that are unmistakably those of a disabled child, one that can't express their emotions verbally, yet they are joyful noises. I check the driver in the rear-view to see if his attitude to us has changed. He seems relaxed, sanguine.

I keep up a steady commentary mixed with questions. *Look, Bear – we're going the same way as the bus! But we're quicker in a cab. Exciting, isn't it?*

This will be the last time I see her until after Christmas. I'm leaving again with a heavy heart. I made the most of our morning together – feeding her porridge oats, yoghurt and chopped apple, brushing her teeth, then afterwards playing songs for her on the guitar. 'Ticket To Ride', 'Days', 'In My Life', 'Wish You Were Here'. During this last tune she stood staring out of the window at the wet street below, seemingly lost in thought.

We encounter traffic. A tailback. As always on these journeys, I'm anxious. If her mood changes and she starts crying or kicking out at the seat in front, we may be ejected, with a repair bill perhaps, and with no hope of getting to the kindergarten on foot. I have my hands clamped tightly over her brown, zip-up winter boots.

So I make a 'tick tock' sound I sometimes do for her, with the tip of the tongue on the roof of my mouth. (This is 'music', of a sort, though hardly the 'Tick Tock' symphony – a basic rhythm, in 4/4 time. A sound like a car indicator, or a metronome, with the accents on the first and third beats of the bar.) It usually makes her laugh, and I want to see if it does this time. What happens next is an event so uncanny, so extraordinary it haunts me on the long train journey back to England. A smile spreads slowly across her lips, and then, without warning, she turns her face and looks me dead straight in the eye. Because of the patchy, low-quality light, and the shadows inside the car, her irises seem almost bronze in colour. Gold, even. In those few frozen seconds, as we hold each other's gaze, both of us smiling, a sort of understanding passes between us. It's such a rare, unexpected, deliberate piece of communication from her that I'm momentarily undone. My eyes prick with tears, yet a feeling of unmitigated happiness – wild happiness – rushes through me. *Oh, Emily. I love you more than my life.*

I want to say this, but the back of the taxi driver's head is inches away. (Although, I have a feeling he wouldn't mind.)

More than anything, I'm struck by how much warmth, trust and affection her eyes transmit. The look is so intelligent, so *human*, and thus freighted with all the subtleties of human communication. Indeed, do I detect a slightly playful, droll, satirical note in her expression? And I suddenly remember the father who said to me, in another lifetime it seems – *it gets so much better when they start to speak, they become people.* He was wrong. I don't need to hear her speak to know she's a person. I don't dream about her speaking any more. I don't need to hear her voice when her expression replies to a question I've asked a thousand times. She has given me her answer, without words. This time I'm certain.

Her look says: *I love you, Daddy.*

And as if to prove it she does something she's never done before. She reaches over and gives me a hug. Snakes her arms around my neck for one brief, eternal moment. Then she rests her head on my shoulder, and we continue the journey in silence.

Further Reading

These are the 11 books that helped me gain a greater understanding of autism. It's a personal, selective list; not meant to be comprehensive.

Berger, Dorita S., *Music Therapy, Sensory Integration and the Autistic Child* (JKP, 2002). 'A unique synthesis of information,' reads the blurb. This excellent book blends science, music therapy vignettes, and practical action plans.

Donvan, John; Zucker, Caren, *In a Different Key: The Story of Autism* (Penguin, 2016). At the time of writing, the best – and most up-to-date – book on the history and science of autism. A fast-paced read, threaded through with personal testimonies from parents of autistic children.

Fernyhough, Charles, *The Baby in the Mirror: A Child's World from Birth to Three* (Granta, 2018). A superb developmental biography of the first three years of a neurotypical child. Especially useful as a comparison text for those parents who have autistic and non-autistic children.

Higashida, Naoki, *The Reason I Jump: One Boy's Voice from the Silence of Autism* (Sceptre, 2013). A revelatory insider account of severe autism, written by a nonverbal Japanese boy using an alphabet grid – a qwerty keyboard drawn on cardboard.

——, *Fall Down 7 Times Get Up 8: A Young Man's Voice from the Silence of Autism* (Sceptre, 2017). The sequel to *The Reason I Jump*, Naoki in his early twenties.

Moor, Julia, *Playing, Laughing and Learning with Children on the Autistic Spectrum* (JKP, 2008). A marvellous practical resource of play ideas for parents and carers.

Moore, Charlotte, *George and Sam* (Penguin, 2012). A richly observed, clear-eyed account of bringing up two profoundly autistic boys.

Normal, Henry, Pell, Angela, *A Normal Family: Everyday Adventures with our Autistic Son* (Two Roads, 2018). Joyful, moving, and very funny.

Park, Clara Claiborne, *The Siege: The First Eight Years of an Autistic Child* (Little, Brown, 1982 [1967]). An exquisitely detailed account of a mother's struggle to cultivate the social, intellectual, and emotional development of her autistic daughter, while refusing to be discouraged at a time when autism was barely understood.

——, *Exiting Nirvana: A Daughter's Life with Autism* (Little, Brown, 2001). The brilliant sequel to *The Siege*. Jessy's life as a young woman.

Silberman, Steve, *NeuroTribes: The Legacy of Autism, and How to Think Smarter About People Who Think Differently* (Allen & Unwin, 2015). Another excellent, and recent, blockbuster history of autism. Highly recommended.

Acknowledgements

I WOULD LIKE to thank my wonderful agent, Oli Munson, who believed in this book from the start, as did my brilliant editor, Oliver Holden-Rea, who gave much encouragement and perceptive advice during the writing process – thank you. I'm also grateful to the excellent team at Bonnier Books.

For their support during the difficult time of writing the book, thanks to Yvonne Enright, Ian Tuton, Amanda Ellis, Ezra Ellis, Riet Chambers, Geoffrey Cook, Tony Ayiotis, Caroline Franks, and Jeff Wood. I'm especially grateful to Jude Cook and Samantha Ellis for their generosity and additional editorial help.

I would also like to thank Kate Mayfield, Ali Mercer for her time and wise words, Cat Andrew for the same, and the Society of Authors for their generous grant. And for divine inspiration: Mark Hollis (1955–2019), Bruno Ganz (1941–2019).

Lastly, I'm grateful to all those who have helped my daughter during her first five years, from the marvellous NHS in the UK, the physiotherapists and occupational therapists, the managers and key workers at the Surbiton nursery to the healthcare professionals in Germany, her ABA therapists, and the one-to-one assistants and staff at her kindergarten – thank you all.

About the Author

JAMES COOK was originally a musician and songwriter for the band Flamingoes. His first book, *Memory Songs* – an exploration of the music that shaped the nineties – was published in 2018. His short fiction has appeared in the anthology *Vagabond Holes*, and he has written about music for the *Guardian* and *Boundless* magazine, among others. He lives in London.

🐦 @jamesbpcook

Useful Websites

Ambitious about Autism: www.ambitiousaboutautism.org.uk

Autistica: www.autistica.org.uk

National Autistic Society: www.autism.org.uk